Walking Into
The Wind

Walking Into
The Wind

---

*Being Healthy With a Chronic
Disease*

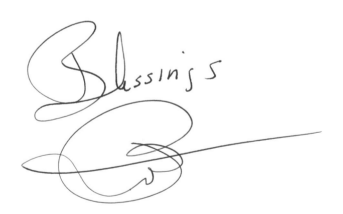

Blessings

Barbra Goodyear Minar

To order additional copies of this book, contact:
Xlibris Corporation
1-888-7-XLIBRIS
www.Xlibris.com
Orders@Xlibris.com

TO GARY
WHO STILL WALKS WITH ME
INTO THE WIND

THE FIRST WIND

June 30, 1960. Laughing and miserable, Gary and I sat on our bed the second night of our honeymoon like two blistered tomatoes, unable to touch each other without wincing. The next morning we continued driving our VW convertible through the Colorado Rockies, not worrying about an innocent sunburn. But that sun released a silent enemy—a wolf that would forever roam my body. In just a few weeks, as we unpacked boxes in our first home on the Air Force base in Cheyenne, Wyoming, fevers, joint swelling, and headaches started. As I walked towards the military hospital, I buried my face in my coat to avoid the stiff, cold wind.

"I see here you're twenty. How long have you been married?" asked Dr. Alfrey, writing notes in my chart—the chart I wasn't allowed to read. "Sometimes it's hard to adjust to married life, especially far away from home. Being a newly-wed can be very stressful." The young blond doctor never looked up. He thinks I'm crazy, I thought. I wanted to disappear from his office, his medical notes, and his nodding head.

The next week my mouth and throat broke out with ulcers. I couldn't eat or sleep. Red flat circles appeared on my toes and fingers.

Soon Gary and I avoided looking at each other. We stopped talking. He went to work. I stayed home, wondering what happened to our honeymoon dreams, our shared secrets, celebrations, and plans. What happened to our new intimacy. What happened to laughter? What happened to my passion for life?

Fatigued and frightened, I hid my discomfort, pushing myself to scrub the bathtub and bake chicken. I substitute-taught at local schools. I worked on a college correspondence course. I'd show my new husband I could cope with married life. I'd show myself. As long as I could work, everything was fine.

Mid-October my temperature soared, and I spent a scrambled week in the base hospital. Late one night Dr. Alfrey took me to an examining room. Without explaining, he attempted a bone marrow test, but failed to penetrate my breast bone with the needle. I was hurt and scared, but I knew I shouldn't cry. It might upset the doctor. He folded his arms and stood by the door in the shadows.

"I've decided we'll fly you to Fitzsimons Army Hospital in Denver in the morning." He paused and cleared his throat. "I suspect you have SLE—Systemic Lupus Erythematosis. " My hands turned cold. I took a deep breath.

"What does that mean?"

"Let me worry about it."

"But don't I need to know?"

"Right now you need some sleep." Dr. Alfrey walked back to the examining table and gently put his large hand on my head. "Is there anything I can do for you?"

"Yes," I whispered. "Tell me if I'm going to get well."

"Of course you are!" He stroked my hair and left the room.

"You won't fly anywhere in this blizzard," said my hospital roommate the next morning. "Listen to the wind."

Plans were changed, and with Gary beside me, an ambulance plowed us through heavy snow. The long trip slipped away as I gave in to my fever. Suddenly I lurched awake. The doors flew open. The ambulance attendants strapped me to a gurney and rushed me into the hospital. I wanted to shout, this is embarrassing! People are looking. But I was silent.

For weeks I swallowed medications and endured tests and examinations. "Hush little baby, don't you cry," sang a black angel in white as she packed me in ice. The sting of the ice burned. I shivered in jerks and tried to stay conscious. I didn't cry.

My mother and father flew out from Mississippi. My mother stayed nearby. Gary drove between Denver and Cheyenne to see me. I meekly did what I was told, and after six strange weeks, I stabilized. I never knew death hung close. Through everything I held on to hope because of the young doctor's promise. I would get well!

Lupus Erythematosus. In 1851 Dr. Pierre Cazenave coined the medical term from the Latin word *lupus*, meaning "wolf", and the

Greek word *erythema* meaning, "to be red." I learned that lupus was a ravenous wolf-like disease of an immune system gone wild. Lupus, kicked off in my case by ultra violet sunrays, made my immune system overactive. I produced abnormal antibodies attacking my own body. The exact cause? Unknown. The prognosis in 1960: five years.

For the next twenty-five years while wrestling with this chronic disease, I had three children, worked part time and finished my college education. I tried to handle my disease by myself, silently biting a stick and enduring. Denial. Denial was my main coping tool.

When lupus violently erupted in 1985, my survival system fell apart. More angry and frightened than ever, I admitted I couldn't tame this wild thing. Finally forced to face the pain and loss, I was surprised by gifts: wisdom and peace, awareness and joy. Now, even with the red wolf growling in my ear, I'm finding out what it *really* means for a human being to be healthy. Through my journal and letters I want to share with you what I discovered from walking into the wind.

MINA

Barbra Goodyear Minar

FEAR'S A FOUR LETTER WORD

Journal
December 17, 1984

Christmas scares me.

I tossed all night. This morning I kept my head under the pillow and my body burrowed in the quilts, trying to catch the dreams still lingering in the sheets. Then I remembered—eight days until Christmas. For twenty-four years some seasons with lupus have been harder than others. This year I can't DO Christmas. I feel like I have boulders tied to my legs. I'm exhausted.

I waited until I heard Gary showering before I moved. The first stretches in the morning made me cry. All my needling joints. I didn't want anyone to see me. Not even Gary. Especially not Gary. When I felt him pass, smelled his pungent aftershave and heard the bedroom door click, I rolled up on the edge of the bed and thought about standing. Standing is hard. But I had to look at myself before anyone else did. I leaned against the bathroom sink and looked in the mirror. Cheeks puffy from prednisone, black circles around my eyes, raised red lesions under my chin, hot sores in my mouth.

Turning my palms up, I looked at flat red circles on my fingers. Signs of lupus. After sticking my hands in warm water to thaw the icy fingers, I put the marked fingertip in my mouth. A storm's coming. The wind's howling. Oh, God, this lupus can't start again. I've had enough surprise attacks from this wolf. Please let this cup pass from me. I want to live!

LIFE AIN'T FAIR

January 3, 1985

Dear Frances,

Thanks for the Christmas card. And, honey, I was in a twit when it came on December 1st. I thought you were a tad over-efficient. But when I found out you'd had back surgery again, I cried.

I wish I had answers for your questions. Seems like we knew a lot more when we graduated from Mrs. Pool's sixth grade than we do now. And remember junior high and high school, talking all night on the phone about the basketball game and school dances and boys? We figured out everything! Funny but the older I get, the less I understand. Some things I simply need to accept. Remember what your Aunt Jeanne used to tell us? "Life ain't fair, girls and life ain't easy. But it's still good."

Thinking about the drunk guy running into your car and your constant back pain for these sixteen years makes me mad all over again. Saying "Life ain't fair" ain't no comfort!

Oh, Frances, I'm scared I might be having another lupus flare. Christmas was hard! Because I'd been hound-dog tired, I put everything off until the school break. Gary insisted on cutting a live tree, and when he got the thing home, it was full of old bird's nest and brown needles. He wired it upright in the den, dirt and all, and tossed some lights around. It was funny, but I was too tired to laugh.

The family made it to the Christmas candlelight service and as usual, I cried through the carols. Christmas morning Gary played Santa in his red hat. I snapped pictures while the big kids (Katherine, seventeen; Jeff, twenty-one; and Steve, twenty-three; and Kathy, Steve's fiancee) ripped open their stockings and gifts.

Oh, honey, seems like everyone came for Christmas and had a great time—but for me Christmas whirled through like a black blur streaked with tinsel. I dragged through the holidays, hiding in the bedroom between events. Head aching, joints swollen, mouth

Barbra Goodyear Minar

full of ulcers. I smiled, trying to look casual, slumped on the kitchen stool stirring gravy or sitting on the kitchen counter drying silverware. The kids helped, but in their young fun they didn't notice I was operating at turtle speed. And really, I didn't want to spoil anyone's Christmas.

I tried to enjoy the moments, but in all honesty I hoped I could keep myself together until the holidays passed. You of all people would understand my fantasies about living on a deserted island.

Oh, Frances, my doctor keeps hinting that I should give up my job at school. But resigning would kill me! I'm going to try and protect myself better from the children (those darling little germ factories). But you know me. How could I direct a preschool without hugging kids? For my New Year's resolution I'm going to take better care of myself. And what do you think about this? Honey, next Christmas I'm going to throw around some holly, order an extra-large pizza with onions and fix hot fudge sundaes.

I promise to get more letters from California to Mississippi this year. And when you feel up to it, please write. I think I'm going to need you, Frances. After years of this up-and-down life, I want God to spare me for a season. But as I rub these swollen knees, it feels like I'm fighting the wind. And I'm afraid.

Love,
Barbra Kay

BARGAINING WITH GHOSTS

Journal
January 18, l985

I'll do everything Dr. Gerber says to do. Except give up my job. It's this fatigue. If only I could shake this fatigue I could press through. Last night Gary came home late from work. Reheating his meat loaf and potatoes and making a green salad seemed like fixing dinner for an army. My tongue was knife sharp. I don't like fixing dinner so late. Gary looked at me and said I should see the doctor. My voice spit like bacon in a hot skillet. "You know I've seen the doctor! All I need is rest."

Yes, rest. I left a messy kitchen and dragged away to my bed. I'll try harder. Eat better. Rest and keep my medicine down. Slumber on, wolf. Oh, if I could only take a hatchet to your throat, I would slaughter you before you wake. Poor Gary. He deserves a better partner. And Katherine deserves a better mother. At seventeen her energy's like a bonfire next to my flickering match. I can't be sick now. I'm sure if I try hard enough, I can stop this thing.

I don't want Gary to know. I'll handle this myself. If anyone knows too much, my freedom could be snatched away, like it was when I had rheumatic fever at four. Stay in bed. Mind the doctor. Swallow the pills. Don't pout. No tears.

One way to keep the wolf asleep is not to mention its name.

Barbra Goodyear Minar

LOSSES IN THE PERSONAL STOCK MARKET

Journal
January 30, 1985

Yesterday I went to see Dr. Gerber with the question, Do I really have to give up my job? I sat in the office as stiff as a broom, remembering what my grandmother said, you can't cry with your chin up. Dr. Gerber came in. My mouth tightened. My throat closed. I lifted my chin and pushed the words out. "Do I have to give up my job?" Dr. Gerber looked at me. He took off his glasses and rubbed his eyes.

"You need to stop working, Barbra."

I bit the insides of my mouth. Tears boiled up. I wanted to bend into my lap and bawl. Instead I nodded my head. Dr. Gerber squeezed my shoulder.

Tonight I told Gary. He was visibly relieved. But it's not settled in me. What about my visions for the school's new library? What about the retreat I planned for the staff? I need purposeful work. The need presses like a hot iron against my chest. All these feelings of sadness, relief, longings, and anger swirl around, making a bitter mix. My soul is full of sweat. But I have no safe place to cry.

I think my heart hurts more than my body.

MINA

ACCEPTING THE WIND

February 5, 1985
Santa Ynez Valley Presbyterian School
1825 Alamo Pintado
Solvang California 93462

My dear families,
As a child, I spent hours lying in the grass watching humid Mississippi clouds. I studied their rapid changes as they shifted their shape being pushed by the wind.

Lupus has become my wind. I've been fighting against its force. But now I must bend and reshape my life by resigning my position as director of the Santa Ynez Valley Presbyterian School.

Because I love serving the staff, families and children of this community, the decision leaves me heavyhearted. But I feel excited about the gifts another director will offer.

The board's first priority is to maintain quality and stability for the staff and children, so I will remain with you until the careful selection of a new director and the transition period have been achieved.

I thank you deeply for your love and support. Now I ask you to watch with expectation the exhilarating forms God will create as we experience shifts from a fresh new wind.

Lovingly,
Barbra Goodyear Minar

TRUTH TELLING

February 27, 1985

Dear Frances,

My heart's in my mouth. My fingers are stopped because if I write the words down they'll make my situation really real. Anyway here goes.

The blood work doesn't lie. My lupus is active. As much as I fought it, I've given up my job, but how I miss the children and young families! In some ways I'm relieved. Working while I leaned against the school walls didn't fool anyone but me. I thought I could grit my teeth, take my pills and press on, but Frances, lying here in bed I'm so exhausted. Even the sheets hurt my skin. I want people to phone, but I'm too tired to talk. I need to be alone, but I'm lonely. Does that make sense?

My body aches. My joints pulse. My face is etched with a red rash. It's hard to breathe. It's hard to think. I feel like I'm vanishing. Slipping out of view of everything alive. People drop cheery notes about getting well but not invitations to lunch. The school's rolling along under another director. The teachers are adjusting, and the children don't know the difference. I feel like I'm stored on my closet shelf. And lupus has shut the door.

Frances, how do you handle Paul's needs? What about your kids? My kids have been through this so many times. My illness scares them. I know it scares Gary. Instead of family, we act like strange roommates, sharing the same kitchen. Everyone moves on cat paws, getting meals, paying bills, folding wash. The silence feels like thunder rolling in the distance, slightly rattling the kitchen windows. You can barely hear it, but sense the storm.

The boys stay busy with their lives away from home, but Katherine's finishing her senior year, and I want to be part of that. Yesterday she plopped on my bed before school and asked if I was any better. Her blue eyes were wet. Her face flushed pink. She looked away as the tears made muddy mascara tracks down her

-MINA

face. I stroked her long fingers saying everything would be all right. But I'm scared. Brushing my teeth is about the biggest thing I can accomplish. Nothing is all right.

Frances, I've got to fight this depression before the wolf drags me off to his den. If I've got to face lupus again, I think this time through I'm going to be brave and tell it like it is. My stomach knots, but I need to shout, *I hate being sick. And I'm afraid!* But I'm not pretending this time. This time through I've got to tell the truth. To open myself to the experience instead of pretending everything is just ducky.

Perhaps I'll learn something that will thicken my soul. But what a risk it is to be honest. What a risk. Will the real me turn out to be a complaining hag? Will my family run away? Every other flare I've tried to carry alone. I didn't feel like it was fair to burden Gary, who's so strong and active, or hamper the kids with a disabled mother. But maybe my illness is a family affair. If I tell my truth, maybe we will grow together. Or maybe like so many families, we will split apart.

I read this by Helen Keller: "Although the world is full of suffering it is full, also, of the overcoming of it." I hate being sick. I want to be an overcomer.

Love,
Barbra Kay

Barbra Goodyear Minar

THE MUD OF GRIEF

Journal
March 14, 1985

Here I am. A waterfall of tears pouring through me. I'm sad, depressed, agitated, angry, furious, irritable, wild, miserable. Sometimes I'm shocked that I'm sick. It's a surprise almost. When I was younger and ill, I used some secret reserve to push through, but now I push and find nothing but quicksand. I'm sinking.

Rains have washed away my house
mud oozes through
the door and pours across
my poor spirit.
Give me Your eyes so I can see how
You can transform me
when winds blow against my life.
if I'll let the bitter go and
let You be God.

HEALTH IS A VERB

April 12, 1985

Dear Frances,

Your letter came at the perfect time. I was lonely, and your encouragement was like water in the desert. I didn't know how thirsty I was for connection.

Your question: Why does God allow pain? Well, once I believed that if I worked hard and was good I could live in sunshine and escape the storms. I know now suffering is part of everyone's life. Sharing the anguish—and the joy—with you helps me be stronger. Maybe it's because I know you understand the struggle.

Question for you. Do you think I could be healthy while I'm sick? Propped up in bed, face numb and head pounding, good health seems impossible. I read recently in the *Los Angeles Times* that people with a good self-image are beautiful, capable and intelligent—healthy.

Well, I've got dark circles under my eyes and a rash on my face—so much for beauty. I'm having a difficult time thinking—finding words and forming sentences. I can't even remember simple facts or people's names—so much for intelligence. I've given up teaching, and I can't even drive to the grocery store—so much for capable. To survive emotionally, I'm going to have to plug in to something deeper.

I miss having something valuable to do. Serving the people I love and doing work I enjoy creates my identity. Lying here I've lost my edges. I feel like my bed is a boat and I'm drifting Frances, I have to work. Maybe then I can get to shore.

I'm risking being more truthful, so I talked to my friend Ann about my work fixation. She urged me to try writing. My chest tightened. I can't write, I argued. I've tried. Even sent some projects out but only got rejection. Ann jumped in with, maybe I need more skills. (Ann never lets up!) Anyway, it turns out a group signed up for the Mount Herman Writer's Conference, and, honey, they plan to take me along—pills, hot pad and all. I could see the set of Gary's jaw when I told him. I know he's afraid I'll get worse. But I know I'll get worse if I don't help myself. It's only for a few days. I can do anything for a few days. I need a new direction. Even if it scares me.

Oh, my friend, how can we be healthy? There must be more to it than fixing our aching bodies and getting back to work. Maybe being healthy means being more human. Crying more, laughing more, smelling rain-washed grass, eating apples right off the tree, looking into the eyes of friends. When we hurt it's hard to believe, but maybe this shadowy "time out" will bring us a gift.

Yesterday I read this letter to God from Betsy, age eight. "Dear God, Are you really invisible or is that just a trick?" Good question!

Love,
Barbra Kay

THE OVERCOMER

Journal
April 28, 1985

> *Fear not that thy life shall come to an end, but*
> *rather fear that it shall never have a beginning.*
> *J. H. Newman.*

I made it through the writer's conference, but I felt so sick when I came home. I didn't want anyone to know how desperately I wanted to fall into my own bed and hide from the wind. So much for my great vow of being honest.

I'm really mixed up about what's being honest and what's being brave. I've been given tons of strokes for not complaining. And that's a good trait, but maybe I've taken it too far.

I have to accept I have lupus.

I think I believe denial is healthier than acceptance. If I act as if my body's fine, maybe I could get away from my dis-ease. Thinking back, I could always talk about lupus if I felt well, but if I felt sick, I slipped into depression.

Yesterday Larry brought donuts by. What a dear friend. He kept knocking around in my kitchen, dumping out donuts and looking for napkins.

Fumbling with my cups he told me to sit down. He was making coffee. He turned toward me, pushing his thick glasses up his Roman nose. His over-large brown eyes floated behind the thick lenses. "Just lead me to the coffee pot," he said. I got the coffee out and he sniffed the grounds and laughed. "You buy the good stuff," he said. "French Roast." I was amazed.

"Yeah," he said, "my eyes are getting worse but my nose is getting better."

It occurred to me that, like Larry, I have a disability. He's legally blind and going to the Braille Institute in Santa Barbara, working

Barbra Goodyear Minar

hard to be an overcomer. Overcomer. Yes, I need to find out how to be an overcomer. But I can't overcome what I won't accept.

If I truly accept my situation, then I'd stop fighting the wind. I've known this in my head for years. If anyone asked I'd say, yes, I have lupus. But I didn't accept it in my gut. Getting into reality could help me be more honest and maybe more assertive about finding help and taking care of myself.

lupus is not my life.

It's part of my life-

but a part I've got to accept. It feels healthy to write this. Yes!

Acceptance.

THE BITTER AND THE SWEET

May 4, 1985

Dearest Katherine,

Oh, little girl! Tonight when I saw you barefoot and pony-tailed, dancing and singing around my bed in your new black prom dress, I laughed and cried. For all the world you looked like you did at four years old, playing dress up, cocking your head to the side and prancing with a high step.

A stone sat in my stomach when I stayed in bed this morning and watched your dad put on his khaki pants and tennis shoes to take you shopping.

"Going to be quite an experience," he said, splashing himself with aftershave like he was getting ready for a date. He stopped and rubbed his forehead. "I've never shopped for a prom dress," he said. I told him to make the day special—take you to Victoria's Cafe for lunch.

After you left I sat in bed and worked on letting go of my disappointment. I imagined you slipping on your high heels and coming out of the dressing room in gown after gown to show your dad. I could see his eyes widening, as he watched his girl-child transformed into a beautiful woman. It'll be hard for him to see you graduate and go to college. After all, you're his baby.

When you came home, he walked into our room and flopped on the bed. With his brow wrinkled into pleats he looked me in the eye. "Are all prom dresses so low in the front?" he asked. "She really grew up!"

Laughing, I ruffled his graying hair. And, funniest thing, the laughter absorbed the last of my disappointment.

Have fun at your prom. Little girl, dance every dance with joy. Wake me up when you get home and tell me every detail.

Kisses,
Mom

Barbra Goodyear Minar

PAIN QUESTIONS

Journal
May 19, 1985

oh, God, where are you? my eyes. am I going blind? my eyes. scleritis—
stabbing pain. dr. winthrop put me on eye drops every two hours. doctor
gerber put me on cytoxan.

i can't read, write, pray.
awake and asleep nightmares swallow me.
maybe I'm being punished.
i am abandoned.
God, take me out of this pain!

-MINA

ILLNESS THAT HEALS

Journal
May 24, 1985

What dark days. Trying to save my eyesight, Ann drove me to Santa Barbara every day to the doctor. With his narrow face serious. Dr. Winthrop took a piercing light and looked deep, deep into my eyes. Thoughts moved through my head like a panicked flock of sheep. What would I do if I went blind?

It was warm last night. Unusually warm, and the spring perfume of grass and night blooming jasmine settled around me as I sat on the deck. My cat hopped into my lap and pressed her black nose into my face and licked her rough little tongue over my cheek. As my fingers ran deep into her thick beige fur, Prissy purred like a one-cat band. Sitting in the quiet, listening to cricket sounds under my asparagus fern and the purring of my cat, I remembered life is more than sight. It's the smell of summer gardenias. It's the touch of a baby's downy hair and a man's rough beard. It's the taste of fresh peaches and my husband's kiss. Yes, even if I went blind, my life would not be over.

Oh, how pain peels away what's important from what is not. As the layers come apart the only things left are relationships and keeping a clean slate with those I love

And, oh yes, living in the moment.

What an odd thought—could illness heal me? In my deep places it's exposing my false visions and misplaced energy. It's challenging my ambitions. Now I have the chance to make new choices. Choices for love. And only love makes an eternal difference. I should have kissed my cat back!

A FRIEND IN MY BOAT

June 7, 1985

Dearest Ann,

Brave friend. You've climbed in the boat with me and have never gotten out. Sometimes when the wind hits the waves, you look seasick with tears standing in your green eyes. Still you're with me. Thanks for the many times you've driven me to the doctor. It's with you I practice honesty. You won't let me escape from myself. You tell me not to be afraid. God has this in His hands.

Thanks for being with me to celebrate when Dr. Winthrop flipped his wild tie and announced the scleritis was under control!

Thanks for reminding me to take responsibility for my life. For keeping friends informed and urging them to pray. For helping me laugh. For bringing in groceries. For encouraging Gary and Katherine. For being servant hands and feet as you quietly unload the dishwasher or wipe off a sticky table.

Thanks for reminding me today on my birthday that I love picnics, movies, singing, popcorn, dancing, parties, jazz, hot fudge sundaes, doves, art museums, good books, new shoes, Far Side jokes, new ideas, balloons, the ocean, hiking, babies, and holy communion. Thanks for reminding me how I love life!

You know I'm scared, Ann, about the chemo treatments, but I'm less afraid because you're going to the hospital with me. Your friendship's the best birthday present I could ever have. All I can say is today Jesus had green eyes.

Love,
Barbra

UNREALISTIC EXPECTATIONS

Journal
June 11, l985

My parents are flying in for Katherine's graduation. Jeff, Steve, and Kathy, my sister and family are all coming. Having everyone here to celebrate Katherine is what I want. I want to do what "regular" families do.

The chemo has helped, but now I'm afflicted with the "curse of a little energy." My body's had a dead motor and, like a poor fisherwoman, I've been pulling and pulling on the rope. Suddenly there's a chug-cough-chug and, by golly, the little boat moves up stream. There's a feeling it's touch-and-go, so I've got to baby her along.

But now that my motor's going, my mind has gone mad. I don't know what to do first, and I can't do very much. The "to do" list is about to swallow me whole. The roses need weeding. The bathrooms need cleaning. The windows need washing. How will I get enough food in? How will I make everyone comfortable? I want to be a normal mom and put a great party together! It's times like these I'm really sick of being sick! I want another body. A healthy body!

I guess in order to be healthy while I'm sick, I've got to deal with the body I've got. I've got to pick out the most important things to do. That wonderful line: Do what's important, not what's urgent.

Okay then—IMPORTANT:
- *Take care of myself.*
- *Get to graduation*
- *Relate to my family*

When these days are over, no one will remember what we ate or where we slept, but only if we laughed and what we said to each other. God, help me keep my motor chugging so I can hug everyone. And help me let the rest go. Oh, yes, the health of letting go!

WHO'S THAT WOMAN WITH THE BROOM?

Journal
June 13, 1985

I'm overwhelmed again. Penny bounced through the back door with a chicken casserole. "Thought you might need this with all your family coming." All afternoon friends brought salads and desserts and a meat loaf and ham in wicker baskets and fancy trays.

Then Francie walked in, brown eyes snapping. "What are you doing with that broom?" She grabbed the broom from my hand and ordered, "You go rest." I obeyed like a robot, lay down and fell asleep listening to the hum of the vacuum. When I got up I discovered Francie had changed sheets in the guest room. Ann had scrubbed my kitchen counters and clipped my old roses. Tonight when Gary brought milk, bread, chips, and soft drinks home, he found a refrigerator cleaned by someone's caring hands.

Why is my heart singing "thank you" and yelling "please stop" in the same breath? What's going on in me? I guess I want to be the one taking care of my home. More than that, I want to be the one helping friends. Giving is wonderful. Giving is powerful. Now I understand, "It is more blessed to give than to receive."

Learning to take and give with my whole heart is another lesson in how to be healthy. There are times for giving and times for receiving. Right now there's a whipping wind buckling my knees, and I need to let someone give me a chair. It takes deep humility to receive with true grace. By receiving the gifts. But letting in love gifts brings health.

GUILT HAS A LONG ROPE

June 19, 1985

Dearest Dad and Hazel,

Oh thank you for coming to bear-hug Katherine in her cap and gown! I'll never forget Dad in my blue checked apron, barbecuing chickens after graduation. And Hazel bringing in bags of lettuce, tomatoes, hamburger, and buns from the store for lunches. Both of you washing dishes, scrubbing pots, shining my copper teapot, saying you were "just tidying up a bit." Your laughter filled the house as you beat me over and over in Hearts. I can tell you I hate that queen of spades!

But sometimes I looked in your faces and saw anxious eyes. And Wednesday when I hugged you goodbye, I saw tears. I don't know how to ease your minds, except to say I'm taking care of myself. Even though I have lupus, I'm learning to be healthy.

Wellness is more than my body working perfectly (although I'm all for that!). Having lupus is like being forced to live in a harsh boarding school. In the past I've been in such anger and denial I didn't learn much. I want things to be different. I have a choice: I can learn to accept my life or not.

Somedays I'm lower than a snake's belly and can't do anything but slide through. But lately I'm reading and thinking a lot about my situation and about my attitude. Maybe I can get my MD (Master of Distress) out of this.

I ache that you're troubled about my illness. As you enter your seventies, it should be my time to support you. Now that you're back in Mississippi, I feel the distance of the miles. But there's no distance between our hearts.

Lovingly,
Barbra Kay

*My mother died when I was twenty-two. My father re-married and Hazel became my mother-in-love in 1962.

Barbra Goodyear Minar

BEING A HUMAN BEING

Journal
June 24, 1985

I'd been feeling so good. Stronger than I had in months. My thoughts swelled like a song. I must have pushed lupus underwater in the river. Held that wolf down so long he drowned. Yeah! I feel so good I know he's dead!

So I pushed my body. Jumped back into denial. Didn't listen to the wind whistling in my ears.

Now I'm flat.

Joints ache, stomach's bloated, weak as a fish on the dock. Would be worth it if I used my energy for something special—like going up in a hot air balloon or dancing in red skirts like a gypsy on top of a table—but I vacuumed the house. Big deal. Who cares anyway?

I see myself in action. I'm Barbra who digs up potatoes, yanks weeds out of her rose garden, spins wild stories for kids, hits a solid tennis backhand, and paints the bedroom ceiling. Lying in bed I feel like I'm waiting to be Barbra. How can I learn Barbra in action is the same Barbra resting?

> *God, teach me that I'm precious sick and well. I'm*
> *valuable simply because*
> *you created me.*

LITTLE PLANS FOR A BIG LIFE

Journal
June 26, 1985

What a morning! I walked across my front lawn and down Quail Valley Road. I walked slowly, listening to the mockingbird in our big sycamore tree. He was singing to celebrate me. I walked a few feet and discovered in the Flishers' bushes a wet spider web. I touched a branch and watched the weaving shimmer like liquid silver. At the Whites' I smelled the sweet honeysuckle and rubbed velvet petals of the red climbing rose braiding itself in the fence.

Suddenly my legs felt boneless. Shaking I walked home and lay down feeling as if I'd walked, not ten minutes, but hiked ten miles. But I did it! I walked!

A few months ago I asked Ann if she thought I was going to die. Guess I asked her because I was afraid to ask myself. I remember her shoulders curved forward as she dropped her hands in her lap. She looked like a small bird with broken wings. "Yes, sometimes I'm afraid of that," she said, turning her face and looking out the window. I felt cold. I reached for her hand.

I'm scared thinking about leaving my body and translating into another form. I can't imagine myself without my body. I've gotten extremely attached to this fragile-clay holder for my soul. When I die, I know I'll be with the One who created me. But I feel overwhelmed when I think about leaving my earth home and my people.

Everyone's earth journey ends in death. Reflecting on my own death is bringing me a gift—challenging me to make choices about using my time and energy. Planning my life is better than letting it happen. I need to be flexible. But planning will help me accomplish some of my dreams and goals. If I don't think about life and death, death could creep up and snatch me before I've lived. I'm looking death in the face so I won't be caught by surprise. I want to live every day with purposeful awareness. I want to see, really see, spiderwebs.

TRUTH TELLING

June 27, 1985

Dear dear Gary,

Tomorrow's our twenty-fifth anniversary. Can you believe it? Sometimes we've had the wind at our back and sometimes in our face. But here we are, still married and going forward. I know some years have been difficult because of my illness. This is one of those years. I know it's hard for us to talk about my limitations. We're silent about our needs for lovemaking. You're afraid I'm too tired, too sick, too delicate to be touched. I'm afraid I'm too unattractive for you to want. We are both too fragile to risk talking. I think we fear if honest words come out, the knitting of our marriage will slide off the needles and everything will unravel. But what we probably need most is to hold each other, to cry, to truth-talk about fear and losses, to make plans and eat more ice cream.

The daydream life of meadow picnics in spring poppies and sweet laughter of happy babies was only half true. We've learned real life isn't all fun. Some of it's painful. Pain can break us apart or pull us together. It can bury us or deepen us. As we meet the future joys and losses, I'll try to be there for you as you've been there for me.

I don't want my lupus to imprison you. My anniversary gift is to commit to you, for richer and poorer, in sickness and in health, to have all the LIFE possible until death do us part.

Love for another twenty-five,
Barbra

-MINA

MAKING MEMORIES

Journal
June 30, 1985

Our anniversary! I rested and rested and rested to be ready. Gary and I drove to Monterey and stayed in the Cosby House, a darling Victorian bed and breakfast. I found it hard to walk far. Each time we tackled an adventure, Gary would drop me off close to the shops, beach, or restaurants, find me a place to sit and then park the car. We managed quite well, and I felt like a sassy girl, flying kites, buying a rope swing, eating giant hot fudge sundaes and salmon at "Alice O's." Between naps it felt great to play.

That night as we lay between soft cotton sheets, Gary ran his hand down my arm. "Remember our wedding day? How the guys pulled the plugs on our car so we couldn't drive off. And how we took all the pictures on our honeymoon without film in the camera? Remember how innocent we were? Remember our sunburns? How I wanted to touch you."

I didn't want to talk about my illness. Not on this weekend. But my anniversary letter had primed the pump, and little by little words stumbled out. Timid words, anxious words. Words and tears. The honesty released the love.

Driving home along the ocean on highway 101, Gary mentioned he may be transferred to Long Beach. Next January. Our conversation stopped. That would mean a move from my home and community. A complete uproot-replant deal. It's hard to put it out of my mind, but I must. I can't think about moving now.

I'm thankful I was strong enough for this trip. The two days away from home were health-giving for us. Thank you, God, for these twenty-five years of growing up. May we grow deeper and closer to you, and to each other.

Barbra Goodyear Minar

THE COACH IN THE WHITE COAT

July 1, 1985

Dear Dr. Gerber

For over nine years you've been my doctor, and these last stormy six months you've grasped my hand as a friend. I deeply appreciate your extra care and interest.

I'm realizing that as a child with rheumatic fever, as a girl with mononucleosis, and as a young woman with lupus, the mysterious gods in the white coats would take my blood and give me pills. The burden of my health was on my doctor. My job was to swallow the pills and not to cry.

Last week when you gently felt my joints, set your glasses on the counter and looked into my face, my eyes filled with tears. You looked into my being, giving me a dose of compassion. When you asked if you could pray for me, my soul rested.

Now I'm realizing that you, medications, and other intervention can support my healing, but only my body can rally to heal itself. I must do more than swallow the pill. My health is up to me. Health of body, mind, and spirit.

Dear Dr. Gerber, you're my Coach in the White Coat. You've encouraged me to exercise, take my medicine, reduce stress, and make peace with my limitations. You've encouraged me to be honest with my family and, more important, be honest with myself. With you as my Coach, I'm committed to take a more active role in my care.

As I think about your quiet gentle way and your attentive listening, I realize what a gifted healer you are. All my doctors have taken my pulse, but few have looked in my eyes and listened to my heart.

Sincerely,
Barbra Minar

THE WAR ISN'T ALWAYS ON FOREIGN SOIL

Journal
July 9, 1985

The big guns have failed. So today I started using a cannon to control this wolf! Ann drove me to the hospital for chemo, both frowning and telling jokes. As I climbed into the hospital bed, I was nervous. Ann was nervous and hovered over the nurse putting the IV into my hand until she was nervous. The medication was hung on a stand to drip in my veins. The nurse patted my pillow, "Don't worry about a thing, Mrs Minar. Just press this button if you need me. Want apple juice or tea?"

I watched the IV for a moment. Swallowing poison all pressed together in a pill doesn't seem too scary. Yes, taking pills are one thing, but putting the stuff straight into my blood stream—well. When the first treatment was done, I went home and slept through frightening drug dreams the rest of the day. Tonight it took me awhile to look in the mirror. Finally I went in the bathroom and flipped on the light . My swollen face was red, but I hadn't grown horns or a beard. I was still me.

Help me be patient, God. Patient with myself, with the healing. There is more chemo to come.

Help me
"fear not"

Barbra Goodyear Minar

THE GIFT OF COMPASSIONATE HEALERS

July 13, 1985

Dear Frances,

I'm recovering from another pulse of cytoxan and solu-medrol. The stuff really works for me—once I recover from the stormy treatment. I feel confident in my doctor. I don't know what I'd do without him. There's certainly an important bond that comes between doctor and patient with chronic problems. When I've talked with other people in Dr. Gerber's waiting room, I see he affects most everyone the same way. I'm blessed to have him. You, on the other hand, have really gotten the run around.

I've been working on what rights (and responsibilities) we have as patients. Sometimes we forget that we're paying the doctors to help us. Sometimes we see them as gods, knowing everything. Sometimes we give them too much power over our lives. Because we need to have a good relationship, we might become afraid to "bother" the doctor with our "small" complaints, choosing only the "big one" to discuss. Or we might be afraid to ask for a second opinion because it might offend the doctor. Sometimes we come to our appointments so confused and sick that depression and frustration replace talking about symptoms and treatments. It's understandable, because we really want to be well—not just coping. And, oh, honey, in our hearts we long to be square dancing, water skiing or travelling to Alaska in a purple hat.

Frances, I encourage you to take more control of your situation. You have the *right* to find a doctor you can work with. Maybe, if you make the change, you won't feel so powerless. It helps me to remember doctors are only people—most of them trying to do their best. But I need to say I'm in charge of myself. I can say "yes" or "no" to treatments or tests or surgeries. And as I partner up with all the medical people, and I do the best I can, I seem to accept my life better. I can watch travelogues and read about Alaska without feeling cheated (I do, however, wear a purple hat).

When I was born, there wasn't a guarantee that I'd get to travel to Alaska or anywhere else. What matters is my existence. Someday we will be free of these temporary "weights" and do some heavenly exploration.

In the meantime, take a big step toward health. Find a doctor who will help you live your life with dignity. You deserve it, Frances. You're the bravest person I know!

Love,
Barbra Kay

P.S. I'm reading a great book by Norman Cousins, *Anatomy of an Illness as Perceived by the Patient.* Cousins was dying from an incredible disease. His doctors at UCLA Hospital had given up hope. Cousins took over his treatment and got well! One of his main "therapies" was laughter. He ordered old movies of W.C. Fields, Groucho Marx and The Three Stooges and watched them around the clock. He made the fantastic discovery that ten minutes of genuine belly laughter gave him two hours or more of painfree sleep. I'm for that!! Read the book and send me a joke.

LOSSES IN COMMON

Journal
July 16, 1985

Phyllis brought her two preschoolers by this morning. Both little fellows were clutching wilting daisies. They handed them to me, talking and grinning, with Jeremy, the four-year-old, explaining how flowers drank water through their stems and these flowers needed drinks right away and I needed to find a jar. Phyllis laughed as they danced around and talked. She was so patient.

When they left, I set the daisies on my bedside table and remembered when my children were small. They had so many needs, and I had so many limitations. Sometimes—when I remember the snap in my voice because six-year-old Steven needed the tire on his bike pumped up, or four-year-old Jeff wanted me to cut windows in his old refrigerator box, or wailing baby Katherine needed me to rock her—I hide my eyes. Some days, some months, it was too much. Did I scar them? Can they recover?

What happens to children with a disabled mother? A mother who (if she washes at all) washes the whites and colored clothes together. Who feels like a crazy woman because of pain and interrupted sleep. Who says, "No, you can't fingerpaint in the kitchen" (I've suppressed their creativity). Who says, "Yes, go turn on the TV" (I've destroyed their imagination). Who can't wait for the children to go to bed at night and groans when she hears them wake too early in the morning (I've made them feel unwanted). I feel guilty. I should have done so much more! I should have been so much more!

In some ways this is the cry of all mothers, I guess. We should have done more. But there are so many holes in my mothering fabric I look like a fish net. I know it was unrealistic, but I wanted everything perfect for my children. Some days getting out of bed and feeding everyone were major miracles.

I'm longing to go with Katherine to her college orientation. I've disappointed her so many times this year. If I rest and rest I know I can make it.

No word from the boys lately. I'm worried about Jeff. His problems with alcohol and drugs send me searching for help. And now his quiet is like a jack-in-the-box with the lid closed. Something is ready to spring up. But Steven's only busy with his life. At his age I already had two babies and wasn't tuned in to my parents' lives at all. Still I ache.

I know I've missed so much. Especially when the wind blew hard against my house. But maybe every reflective parent would say the same. I'm realizing many of my losses are common losses in everyone's life.

GOOD ENOUGH MOTHER

July 17, 1985

Dearest Steven,

Thanks for the long newsy phone call. I was feeling lonely for a connection with you. There's something extraordinary about one's first child that lodges in a parent's bones forever. Someday I hope you and Kathy will have this fantastic experience.

You see, the baby reshapes the lovers who helped shape the baby. And when that infant takes his first breath, all you ever knew of love is suddenly challenged. Turned inside out like your pants pocket, you dump all you have and find you need and want to give more—more love, more time, more money, more patience, more wisdom. The baby begins teaching the parents everything—(whether you wanted to know it or not).

Steve, many people have children so someone will love them. But it turns out the parent needs to be a hundred percent unconditional lover—learning to discipline, setting boundaries, studying the child's personality, on and on.

Having you share your childhood memories is helping me sort out my history. I told Rebecca about my parenting failures the other day. After I read the list from my journal she lowered her head and furrowed her brow. Then she leaned across my bed, adjusted her glasses and looked hard into my eyes. I thought she was going to tell me the worst.

"Well, Barbra, I think every mother in the world could make a list like that one." Then she leaned back and laughed. "We are all disabled mothers. Trying to raise another human being is almost impossible. Only God can raise a child." I love you, my son. Thanks for letting me know that even though I'm disabled like all the rest, I am a "good enough mother." You've relieved my heart.

Love from your first friend,
Mom

-MINA

GIFTS FROM A DISABLED MOM

Journal
July 20, 1985

Last night Maria's sister Leah called me from Tennessee. She's six weeks pregnant and has SLE. Her voice high-pitched like a little girl's, she skirted around asking polite questions. Then pow! How'd you do it, she wanted to know. "Even though my doctor's unhappy, I'm having this baby. I'm not so scared about my health. Can I ask you a personal question?" Her voiced dropped to a whisper. "I just want to know—did your kids suffer because you have lupus?"

As we talked I remembered how lupus wrestles with a pregnancy sometimes—like it did the nine months with my Katherine. And how it wrestles you for the good moments with your child. I knew she'd probably have some rough days—but also joy days.

"It's easy for me to bash myself," I said, "about my mothering failures, not being able to hike in the sun, go swimming or boating. Not being able to make all-day school field trips. For having to nap instead of roller skating. It's not easy for any mother. But there are some special things children gain from a 'quiet' mother."

"Like what?" asked Leah. "I need a list."

I jotted some ideas down as we talked.

- *They knew I was nearby listening, talking, watching them play.*
- *They loved sitting with me in bed after school, telling me about their day.*
- *They learned to cook, use the washing machine, dryer, and vacuum cleaner, creating great self-confidence.*
- *They learned to help each other. Also to work out their own disagreements.*
- *They learned to live with someone whose energy is a gift.*

Barbra Goodyear Minar

- They became aware that disabled people are not "odd balls" but simply people with challenges.
- They developed a sensitivity to people with problems.

"The negatives are obvious," I told Leah, "but there are also many positives. I think children living with a disabled parent can become more self-reliant, kinder, and more aware."

"I want to believe you," said Leah. "I want to believe I can be a good mom."

"Your baby doesn't need a perfect mom," I told her. "Your baby needs you. A good enough mom. Call me anytime. And take good care of yourself."

We hung up. My eyes flooded. I am a disabled mother. And that's O.K.

ADJUSTING THE LENS

Journal
July 25, 1985

Katherine and I made it to Sacramento State. Mission accomplished! I'm in bed now but glad I spilled my energy on this trip. I'm grounded better, seeing where my baby bird will nest. The campus of lush trees, the dorms, lecture halls, and labs, the enormous library, piles of bikes and backpacks. The glowing young faces, talking, walking, lounging, romancing, and, oh yes, studying, etched themselves in me.

I had two experiences going on at once. First, joy with my daughter. Watching as her new environment took its first frightful and wonderful sweep; listening as she said, "Do I look all right, should I be a business major, did you see that cute guy, where do I cash a check?"

At the same time I felt crushed, being on campus with energetic, vital people. The professors and parents and students felt strong, directed, invincible—full of goals. My main goal was to find a place to sit down.

"Go on, Katherine," I said gratefully. "Meet me back here before lunch." I collapsed on a wooden bench. As I watched the people rushing by, they made a powerful river. I was sitting on the bank. I didn't even have enough energy to cut bait and fish. Everyone I saw was pulling in the big ones. Probably they were rocket scientists, brilliant novelists, deep philosophers, or promising students—adding something positive to life.

As the fantastic people-parade went by, something black started gobbling at my insides. Slumping against the bench, I was too worn out to fan myself in the heat. Then a girl in a blue wheelchair pushed herself along the sidewalk. A red backpack was strapped to the chair and her bumper sticker said, "Bloom where you're planted."

Thank you, God, for that messenger. She busted me out of my pity prison. My life isn't over because I have limits. I'm going to start writing. Even if the risk scares me. Even if I'm too tired to sit at my desk.

Barbra Goodyear Minar

Even if I have to tackle the computer. Even if I'm not very good at word-working.

I am going to start writing. Even if I have to write in bed. I'm going to bloom where I'm planted.

-MINA

MINI-SERVICE

July 27, 1985

Dear Frances,

I loved the jokes you sent. What about this:

Three nurses died and met Saint Peter at the pearly gates. He asked the first one,"What did you do on earth?"

"I was a nurse in ICU."

"Wonderful, wonderful," said Saint Peter. "Come right in! What did you do on earth?" he asked the second nurse.

"I was a nurse in a pediatric hospital."

"Wonderful, wonderful," said Saint Peter. "Come right in! And what did you do on earth?" he asked the third nurse.

"I was a nurse for an insurance company."

"Wonderful, wonderful," said Saint Peter. "Come right in for forty-eight hours." HA!

Your idea of writing down medical information directly on our calendars is great. Maybe we'll see patterns emerge that could add pieces to our puzzle. I'm doing it and will take the info with me to my next appointment.

Oh, honey, I understand your depression, and I honor your battle. Last week I felt like the sun went out. Rebecca called. I didn't want to talk. Ann came by. I didn't even comb my hair. Trying to discover the cause seemed fruitless. I was depressed about everything. The way I felt, the way I looked, my marriage, my mothering, my loss of work, my lack of energy. When I heard my friend Lana is going hiking with her husband into the Grand Canyon in October, I suddenly found myself waving a "poor me" flag.

I'm often thrown in the boxing ring with depression. I'm looking for punches to throw at my opponent. And I'd really like a knockout once and for all—bells ringing, my arm lifted by the ref announcing, "Barbra, the all-time winner." Oh, YES, Honey! But I think with my situation I'll be back in the ring over and over. I need more training to learn how to cope with stress, disappointments, and fears. Then I can fight the depression better and move on.

The raw wind of lupus this year has brought with it deep sadness. I've had trouble thinking and talking. Now for a word-lover like me that's devastating. Perhaps for my family and friends it's a relief (a little humor there)! Communication is a big part of "me." Stressing about my thinking blows my thoughts and words farther away. And pushes my attempt to write out the window. Then I stir my pity-pot and eat the muck I cook up. Believe me! It's not a healthy way to live!

So I thought, Barbra, you *need* to serve others. I could give mini-services. I'm zeroing in on a few house-bound folks. Phone them just to listen, to tell jokes, to care.

Also I had this "big writing" idea, but with my mind shorting out I feel stuck. Maybe I could have a "little writing" idea. Little but mighty. Since my words are in short supply, I'm going to start zipping off a few one-line postcards to people who are "off the road."

Another thing I can do is listen. Listening doesn't take much energy, but it's a great gift to give. Most people can talk out their problems if someone will listen.

There are so many people coping with difficulties. I think when God hands out gold medals, we'll be surprised at the hidden "bravehearts" he rewards. I'm going to look for bravehearts to serve. And this will help me fight my own depression.

Really these mini-services are selfishly for me—to help me keep healthy. You know, good hearty spiritual spinach instead of muck from that pity-pot.

Love,
Barbra Kay

PUSHING OUT

July 29, 1985

Dear Beverly,
I'm thrilled to be coming to Tahoe. Thankfully, yesterday I finished a course of chemo. I should be stronger when I see you on the sixth. Oh joy! We can talk and talk.

Blessings,
Barbra

LIVING IN THE NOW

Journal
August 6, 1985

This must be a dream—I'm in Beverly's guest room. I planned to relish this time away. But my skeleton has turned to sand. My stomach roars hungry but rejects all food. Maybe the trip was too ambitious. I'm boxing with depression. What can I do to be healthy? What?

Enjoy the moments. Enjoy the grace gifts of beauty.

I'm in a massive pine four-poster feather bed. I feel like I'm nestled in a cloud. The pine planks of the cathedral ceiling butt into one massive pine log. Cross beams are split logs. Walls are padded fabric of maroon-red cherries and green leaves. Hand painted cherries sprinkle the bathroom tile. The floor, made of wide pine planks, is the color of honey. A wall of native gray-green stone backs a wood stove with gleaming brass trim. Besides the bed, four other pieces of antique furniture are in the room: pine desk, small bedside table, and a marvelous deep wing chair with side tray table, painted with roses and green ribbon. From the tall narrow windows I can see Lake Tahoe, sun glints dancing on the blue. Pines and redwoods, growing close to the house, lay branches like long green arms against the window. Between the limbs blow spiders' weavings, flexible and unthreatened.

A Steller's jay looks in at me from his world. He cocks his head, probably wondering if I'm caged behind glass.

How could he know I'm peaceful? Living. Looking. Seeing. How could he know? I am free!

CHOOSING TODAY

Journal
August 5, 1985

I was awake well before the sun struck across the room and washed my face. Last night Katherine called, saying Jeff is home and needs help. I slept little. My mind rolled between dreams and prayers. God, what can we do for him? What should we do for him? If only I'd been a better mother. If only I'd tackled the signs of his addiction more aggressively. If only I had more wisdom.

I left the solitude of Bev's place. I went into torment.

I got up for tea and climbed back in bed. The wind whipped the lake, chopping it into blue and white sections. My windows were open and it was cold, but I bundled up in blankets and leaned back on huge soft pillows. Then I made a choice. Not to miss being here. To live in the moment. And deal with tomorrow tomorrow.

Lunch turned into hours of sharing as Bev and I spread out the questions of our hearts. Questions of faith. Questions about loving our men. Questions about guiding and delighting and fearing for our children. Because of our friendship, we created a transparent trusting place. A rare place.

Around three I sat on the redwood porch. The sky was full of drifty thin clouds. Curling slightly at the edges, they hung in the blue like a veil. Somehow they didn't seem too serious about being clouds—lazy like. My feet rested on a low stone wall shaded by thick evergreen trees. The pungent smell of pine and spruce and redwoods perfumed the afternoon. There are big holes crafted in the deck for three large redwoods. Between the wall and the lake area stood a hedge of trees. I could see the lake from this secret spot, but no one could see me

I drank mint tea and wished I could sit in the sun—get hot and tan. Leap in the lake off the pier for a shivering swim and lay my long self back on the warm boards to soak up more sun. I remembered how the warm rays felt when I was sixteen. Now at forty-five and getting

Barbra Goodyear Minar

well, I chose not to inflame the wolf; to content myself hidden in the shade.

On my way inside I met two cheerful women shaking rugs at the back door. The rooms were filled with fresh flowers and clean sheets and puffed pillows and scrubbed sinks. A dozen red roses and baby's breath, blue bachelor buttons and tiny yellow button mums were mixed in several vases. Blue and yellow iris stood like princesses on the game table.

The smell of two gardenias floated in the guest room where I packed. Many grateful people will rest in this womb-like space. And enjoy the greatest gift in this house, Beverly herself. Blessings and peace to all of you who dream here after me.

I am anxious about going home.

I am grateful I was able to come.

WRESTLED FROM THE PEACE

August 15, 1985

Dear Bev,

I treasure the peace from your home. I came back to a hornet's nest, and things haven't stopped buzzing. Every family member hurts from the poison of addiction seeping through our minds; stinging us in unexpected attacks. I am trying to find the ways I am addicted to fixing my son. Alanon is helping. I have deep inner work to do.

Bev, I've thought about the rich talks we had. You're like a crystal glass; clear honesty reflecting both your creative personality and process. I'll always treasure your openness. Working with our questions is important, and now I'm struggling with "What is my responsibility?" Responsibility to Gary, myself, children, friends, parents, community, church. The list is endless really. The burning question today is, "What am I responsible for concerning Jeff?" And I'll be healthier when I can answer that. Sometimes my mind seems like the white head of a dandelion. I make a decision. Then a gust of wind hits, and my thoughts float off scattering everywhere. Now I understand the old saying, "I can't get ahold of myself."

I'm grateful I've stored a bit of your place in my soul. I'm going to need to retreat there. I fear the pain in the days ahead. Not only the pain of my disease, but soul pain that strangles me from within about my young son. I don't want to be like the frog plopped on the stove in a pan of hot water—sitting and sitting—adjusting and adjusting—until the water's boiling and she's cooked. I need breakthroughs and change. And the only person I can change is me.

Please stay in touch, and let my thanks warm you. I didn't miss a detail of your kindness.

Lovingly,
Barbra

CUTTING THE APRON STRINGS

September 10, 1985

My dearest Kath,
How are things going this week at school? My love, when I hear you cry over the phone, I'm wondering what the tears are really about. From the time you were tiny, you've always been my get-up-and-go kid. Spend the nights away from home—no problem. Off to camp—no problem. Being away at college, however, is another deal. A life structure change. Hang in there.

Your dad and I are working with Jeff. We're going to Dr. Root for counseling, and Jeff's enrolled in Santa Barbara City College. I know you worry about him. We're all in this together, but Jeff's choices are in his hands. Pray for him and work on letting go.

I fear some of your sadness has to do with me. I do have an illness, but that's in my boat, and I'm learning new ways to sail. Your being home won't stop lupus from hanging around. I promise I'll let you know of any life threatening development. In the meantime, live free!

I went to Dr. Gerber yesterday, and although this fatigue hangs on like a bulldog, my lab work looked stable. Now rest about me, little girl. And experience college to the fullest. The unfamiliar will look familiar as the months pass.

Love you,
Mom

P.S. We'll call you Sunday night. Kisses!!

-MINA

CHAOS AND HOPE

Journal
September 16, 1985

Jeff has dropped out of school. Today he cried with me. I prompted him to be admitted to Pinecrest Hospital for detox and treatment. Eyes red, face gray, he nodded a pain-filled yes. I grabbed him and hugged his limp body. He put his heavy head on my shoulder, and I told him we'd support him; the whole family could be involved at Pinecrest.

Bitter wind whistles a thousand questions and a thousand fears through me. I'm full of hope, yet afraid to hope. I pray he is still willing to go in the morning. God, heal us. Tomorrow is Jeff's twenty-second birthday.

ONE BODY, ONE MIND, ONE SPIRIT

Journal
September 29, 1985

> *You were tired out by the length of your road*
> *Yet you did not say, 'It is hopeless.'*
> *You found renewed strength*
> *Therefore you did not faint.* [1]

God, you know everything about me. How weak I feel. How scared I feel when I look at my son. How scared I feel when I look at the sore, red circles on my fingertips. How my face goes numb when I see the struggle in this hospital. I wonder about the link between my body and my emotions. I would have gotten the answer right on a test. "Oh, yes, emotional health and physical health are a pair of twins." Now I'm knowing it in my soul. But what do I do?

When I look at my son's dark thick brows and hair, chiseled features, full lips, I see a young man brimming with promise. Until he's physically hurt. Until he's in trouble. Then I see a baby, a toddler, a small boy. He needs food. He needs his yellow blanket. He needs love. He needs—he needs—he needs me. The pictures run together. Boy or man? The definition slides back and forth, depending on if the ice in his world gets thin and cracks.

What is my responsibility? What? Like a tornado, demands whirl in my mother-stomach. I never got him launched. Take him back in the nest and feed him some more. Strengthen his wings. Try again. When he falls from the sky I feel guilty. Because the food I've fed him didn't grow him. And the flying lessons I've taught him didn't launch him. Yes, I feel guilty—and crazy.

But, God, the tips of my fingers are red and sore. I'm tired. In my deep places I'm tired. I need to do this a different way, or he can't be healthy. I can't be healthy.

Tonight at the hospital group meeting, a woman with silver hair told the story about her daughter. Beautiful black-haired Julie on the street using drugs and used by men. "What happened?" asked her mother. "What happened to her life. And my life?" With red eyes and nose running she looked at us, one by one. Her flooding dark eyes caught mine and suddenly I knew. She felt like I felt. I swallowed tears burning my throat. Swallowing tears isn't healthy, God. I held them through the meeting. I held them the forty miles home. I've held them for a lifetime. Here they come. Here they come. Catch them, all, and put them in your bottle. Please, someone kiss my red fingertips.

WHOSE SKIN DO I LIVE IN?

Journal
October 1, l985

I feel like a part of myself is waking up. I have that tingling sensation like when my foot's gone to sleep. I move it and the blood flows back. It hurts, but I let the hurt come. I know it's a good thing for my body. I'm becoming more aware. And the sensation hurts. I have done things I ought not to have done. With the very best of intentions. I have a boundary problem with my son. I don't know where our skins, our minds, our souls start and stop. I wanted him to take life in his teeth. But he did not. So I went out of my body into his to help him. When he got in trouble and was hurt, I was hurt. When he got a job and was happy, I was happy. When he lost his job and was sad, I was sad. The emotions of his life drive my life, as surely as if I had a bit in my mouth and handed him the reins. And I'm galloping out of control while he shouts and cries.

This is health. I'm beginning to take my feeling back in my own skin—and it hurts.

BREAD CRUST AND THE REAL TRUTH

Journal
October 11, 1985

Yesterday Suzanne turned fifty, so I asked her over for lunch. She started talking about the shock of being middle-aged. Then her voice trailed off. The corners of her small mouth turned down and she looked old. Gravity pulling at the freckled skin of her cheeks and neck. Gray streaking her red hair. Suddenly she bent across her red "special person" plate and began pulling the crust off her ham sandwich.

"I don't have to eat this any more. I hate crust. I'm not gonna eat this any more!" Her voice became boisterous. "No matter what anyone says!" She looked about seven-years-old, eyes sparkling, nose in the air. As she made a pile of crust on her napkin, Suzanne started laughing. Then she folded her arms. She looked so young and strong I promptly ripped the crust off my sandwich.

What a process awareness is. And sometimes I don't move toward change because I've gotten too invested in what I thought was right. What I thought was truth. Goodness! I can't do something different. I'd be admitting there's a better mouse trap than the one I depended on all this time! My body tingles all over. It hurts. But it's so good.

Be patient, Barbra. It took a long time to form the belief that you had to eat your bread crust. Parents and school and friends and doctors told you, be a good American and eat your crust. You must answer all your phone calls and letters. And write thank you notes within one week. You must get all the work done before you can play. You must. You must. And how have I interpreted all the messages I've received? How have I built "my personal truth?" I have some major work ahead if I'm going to take back my boundaries. Let Jeff live in his skin, consequences and all. And let me live in my skin, consequences and all.

I'm reading Paul Tournier's <u>The Meaning of Persons</u>. He says it so well.

> *We might say that progress in our knowledge of ourselves is*
> *progress from uneasiness to uneasiness . . . Here and there we*

Barbra Goodyear Minar

may catch a gleam of light, a reflection of it, just at those
humbling moments when we perceive that we are not what
we thought we were. [2]

All this work is healthy. I'm in pain and getting well in my soul. And,
I pray, so is Jeff.

MOTHER LOVE

October 13, 1985

Dearest Jeff,

We have come a long, long way. This month I'm learning. It's as if I have been following you on a swaying rope bridge. And suddenly I've been told I have no business on this bridge; to get off and walk my own path.

I've learned that many things I did to help you have actually harmed you—and me. I'm afraid—so I've tried to control and "fix" your life.

Please forgive my outbursts of anger, my manipulation. I need to learn what I am responsible for and let the rest go. My only hope is to find God and entrust our lives to Him. I need to hang the serenity prayer inside my head and practice it before I swing my weight around like a tragedian. You are not my enemy. You are my beloved son. Your illness causes me great grief, but only you can be the warrior of your battle. I must pull out of your war and fight the enemies in my own camp.

Wrestling with shadows makes me sick. I must step into the light and wrestle face to face with change. I must come away from the window where I watch everything you do. I must turn to my own work. I must take back my emotional life. I must walk deeper into my spiritual life. Then when I turn back to you, perhaps you'll see the face of a strong woman who loves herself and loves you better.

I'm trading in control for prayers. One day I pray we can both sing this Psalm.

> Thou hast turned for me my mourning into dancing;
> Thou hast loosed my sackcloth and girded me with gladness;
> That my soul may sing praise to Thee, and not be silent.
> O Lord, my God, I will give thanks to Thee forever. [3]

I Love us,
Mother

THE GIFT OF INNER HEALING

Journal
October 15, 1985

Waiting at Pinecrest for an Alanon women's group to start, I'm thankful for paper and pen so I can secretly spill out my agony, anger, and questions. Last night our counselor asked me, "Do you have any frustrations you'd like to discuss?"

I felt like I was holding back a scream. There was this scream. Sitting in my chest while I talked in a rational tone.

"I am concerned about the best way to help myself make healthy changes," I said. Suddenly, I was aware that my lips were numb, as if I'd had a shot of novocaine. The feeling spread across my face. Soon my scalp was numb.

I wanted out of the pain.

I see I have to go into the pain for my learning. IN. Not over. IN. Not around. If I go in, I learn. I get wider and deeper. My journey is more solid. Full of integrity for eternal solutions and soul growth. So I am in this place. Not to cure Jeff, but to cure myself. To get well I not only need to learn a lot, but I also need to unlearn a lot.

Somewhere I learned being stoic was good. Being stoic put others first and myself last. I had the best of intentions. But being stoic isn't honest. I end up a depressed victim. Now I see why my feet are stuck on this fly paper. Oh, what a trap. If I'm going to escape, I will have to change. Yes, I can be loving but honest. I feel like Debbie fighting with her anorexia. I see her so thin she's almost translucent. I know she's starving. It's so obvious to me she's dying. But she sees no alternative. She knows she's fat. Her stomach feels full if she takes one bite of food. My focus on Jeff feels right, but I'm starving. I have to eat food from my own plate. Working on someone else's life may be easier than working on my own.

I'm glad I'm discovering my responsibility. I am glad the curtains are being ripped down from my windows. The doors being thrown wide open. The roof being torn off shingle by shingle. But the light is too blinding all at once. I pray, God, hide me under the shadow of your wing.

THE PROOF

October 30, 1985

Dear Frances,

Forgive me for not writing, but my life's been swirling. I've been submerged in soul pain. I'm exhausted from the stress of Jeff's hospitalization for addiction problems. Oh, honey, I had it figured out! Just get that kid in a hospital, let the doctors and counselors fix him up, and he'll be on the road. Wrong.

What's happened is that I'm learning more about myself. If I ever needed proof that my emotional life and my physical life are linked, I've got it.

My blood pressure went up. My blood work came back screwy. My joints and head ache, and I feel like I've been hit by a train. Perhaps I have.

Looking closely at the picture, I think I'm embarrassed my emotions are so connected to my physical experience. I learned that a good girl should keep a stiff upper lip, stay calm, cool, and collected. A physical expression of an internal problem shows a character flaw—weakness.

Now I'm thinking that's a bunch of hooey. My body, reacting to its environment, is saying, "Yes, I'm fully aware that things are crazy. Make some changes, ya' hear?!" Maybe my body is healthier than I thought. Giving me signals constantly. And I should pay attention.

Frances, try something with me. Put your emotional stresses—good or bad—on your daily calendar. See if there's any connection with your physical life. I've started tracking things, and it seems three days to one week after stress, my body announces, "I've had it!" Write me back with your results.

Keep us all in your thoughts. We have a long windy journey to make. Honey, life is glorious, but life is also dangerous.

Love,
Barbra Kay

P.S. Maybe we ought to get a huge calendar and write not only physical and emotional experiences, but the simple gifts of our daily life.

DAILY GRACES

Journal
November 2, 1985

After all my rejections, I got my first tiny writing assignment—to do a devotional for <u>The Word in Season</u>. The news broke through the laboring over my son and focused me back on my own life. I feel gladness returning.

I've been reading Tim Hansel's book, <u>You Gotta Keep Dancin'</u>. His personal journey, living with continual physical pain from a broken back, grips me. He really exposes his emotions and unfolds how God worked with him to discover joy even in his agony. He learned to appreciate daily graces.

> *I began to relish small, daily, simple things—*
> *and realized at a depth that never seemed possible that all of*
> *life was sacred. There were moments, though sporadic and far*
> *apart, when I began to understand that life wasn't over for*
> *me—but perhaps was just beginning.[4]*

I think Hansel's right. I need to practice this art. The art of being where I am and enjoying the sacred in the simple.

Today I stood at the sink and washed the breakfast dishes. My hands moved in an ancient rhythm like women washing before me at enamel sinks, wooden buckets, and cold rivers. Dipping in and out, washing around and around. Warm water pouring through my fingers. Soap bubbles dripping off the back of my hands. I gazed out the kitchen window past the redwood we planted in memory of Grandmother Goodyear to see how much taller the pines had grown and if the red flag on the mailbox was visible through the trees. It felt soothing to wash the dishes. It was a gift.

If I look for grace gifts, each day they are here. I simply need to open my mind and eyes. I'll make a list of the simple things around me—so precious—so unsung. My French doors looking out to the oak tree, my bed and pillows, the glass of cold water on my table, my reading glasses, my stack of books, paper, and fine-tip pens. Cheddar cheese and green apples in my kitchen. My phone to the outside world.

Naming is important. Naming these gifts one by one gives them power to lift me into gratefulness. Oh, God, I am grateful for these little sacred graces.

Barbra Goodyear Minar

VANISHING FRIENDS

Journal
November 4, 1985

Well, I picked up the phone this morning and called Gloria. I miss her. We used to meet often for coffee, talk about our lives and the world. I think she disappeared from my life when I got sick last December. She had offered to drive me to Linda's Christmas party. I said I couldn't go because I was having a lupus flare, and I remember her voice got gravelly like it does when she's tearful. Said she had to go. She was already late.

"I hope you feel better," she said. "Goodbye."

Since then she's dropped me from her life. Like the few other times I've called, today her voice was polite but chilly. Today I finally said goodbye. My stomach hurt. I lifted my chin but the tears squeezed out anyway. Goodbye.

There are many losses connected with chronic illness. I've been able to let go of some, but the loss of friends makes a deep cut. Friends who leave the relationship because I am sick. Afraid I'll be a burden. Afraid they'll say the wrong thing. Afraid I might die and they'll hurt. Afraid of my reminder, they too are vulnerable to accidents and illness and death.

If only they knew no one can take their place in my life. But for my own health I must let them go without any bitterness. And if they resolve their fears, I'll be ready to say "Hello, friend."

THE SCHOOL OF THE SPIRIT

Journal
November 12, 1985

God, suffering seems to go on and on. I plug my ears to block the howling of the wolf. I am totally silenced. I have no words. No writing. No drawing. No vision. I have no energy. All I envisioned myself to be—whole woman, caring wife, solid mother, dutiful daughter, firm friend, I am not. When I'm depressed it feels impossible to do the things that will lift my life. I can't sleep, I can't eat, I can't laugh. I hide curled up. Face in my pillow. Eyes dry.

My old ways of coping aren't working. I have been more diligent about some things. I've turned to face the wind.

- *Informing myself about medical issues concerning my disease.*
- *Learning how to talk with the doctors.*
- *Taking responsibility for my body.*
- *Understanding the link of my emotions to my physical life.*
- *Trying to change harmful attitudes and behaviors.*
- *Seeking to live one day at a time.*

All this is good but my efforts alone are not enough. What more can I do?

I've come to believe—to believe God can restore me to sanity if I surrender to Him. I want to touch rock in my spiritual life.

Oh, Maker of me. Lift me up and carry me into the pool and I can be healed.

I hear you ask, "Do you want to be healed?"

I answer, "Yes, yes!"

"Then take up your pallet and walk," you say.

There's more to healing than actions. You honor my choice. I say,

"Yes", roll up my pallet, and put it on my shoulders. But you put your hand on my head in blessing, so I can walk. Walk with you.

My body, holy carrier of my soul and spirit, is only temporary. I'll tend it and help it be as strong as it can be. But my healthy spiritual life will go on forever.

Walking Into The Wind

THANKSGIVING HEALING

Journal
November 23, 1985

Thank goodness we got Steven home for Thanksgiving with his leg in that machine and his knee constantly being bent day and night. Total knee reconstruction from a skiing accident. For all his twenty-four-years and six-foot frame, tonight he wore his ten-year-old face. When we helped him to the couch, he moaned, "I wonder if I let the doctors do the right thing. At least I could walk before this."

Thanksgiving would feel incomplete without Steven. He's in the right place, because Thanksgiving is a healing day. I remember the Thanksgivings on my grandparents' Kansas wheat farm and also at my childhood home in Mississippi. That day we put away the year's sadness, frustration, and worry. Laughter and thankfulness and joy took their place at the feast.

The cooking rituals passed down through the women. Setting the table with Grandmother's handpainted dishes and the special green basket filled with Indian corn and apples and red and yellow leaves. Choosing and stuffing and basting and cooking and slicing the turkey. Mixing the smells of that tender bird with cranberry and yeast breads and green beans with almonds and mashed potatoes awash with butter and thick gravy with onion and giblets and home-made pickles. Baking chocolate cakes and pecan and apple and lemon pies and brownies and chocolate chip cookies. No one ate breakfast. They let the smells tease them and listened to their stomachs growl. People snuck through the kitchen, lifting steaming pot lids, stealing turkey bits. Everyone helped at the last minute. Mashing potatoes, stirring the gravy, slicing the bread, carrying the dishes to the table. Then all gathered around, with thankfulness for life.

Coming to the table made us feel like a part of the community. Old, young, well, or sick—made no difference when we were at the table giving thanks and eating in splendor. After dinner, too full to move, we would eat dessert. The children drank a splash of strong coffee

Barbra Goodyear Minar

in their cup of cream and sugar, and with elbows on the table, listened to the adults tell their stories.

There's something healthy about ritual and traditions. I remember the year Uncle Jack was so sick. He lay on the living room couch all morning, wheezing and looking gray, but when dinner was served he came to the table the most thankful of us all—he said so in his prayer. And it made Grandmother cry.

This year I couldn't duplicate Grandmother's lavish meal, but by paring down things and asking everyone for help, I was able to continue the tradition. We ended with coffee, pecan pie and family stories. And as I laughed in thankfulness and joy with my children, husband, and friends, the sadness, frustration, and worries of the year fell away. I felt whole and very rich. And I could see by Steven's bright eyes he was healing.

SOUL HEALING

Journal
November 25, 1985

Today Mother would have been sixty-nine. She died too young at forty-six. I'm grateful she left me a legacy of love and laughter and faith. As I walk deeper into my need for God, I feel the deep pull of my mother and grandmother and great grandmothers. I am English, Scotch-Irish, German, and French. A European mutt.

For centuries my family stands marked by the cross. Christians. They prayed faith for their children and their children's children. For me before I was conceived. I, too, was marked. And so my blood and bones cry with a deep longing from my family roots to enter into the mystery of God through Christ. To embrace the Old Testament chosen Jews and accept my graft into God's family. Is that why the ageless Psalms cradle me, rock me?

You who made the wind hold me in your mystery. Yes, rock me, God, in your spirit. And I will be content. Teach me about the deep life and I will be healed in the deep places.

FRIEND BUILDING

November 30, 1985

Dear Rebecca,

Today when you said you felt sad you can't do anything for me, I wanted to slap my legs and laugh. You of all people have given me gift upon holy gift. Your commitment to meet with me every Thursday is like a promise of fresh spring rain.

How can I thank you for your *being*. I can't imagine my life without you in it. It seems like when we started talking eight years ago, we each brought a nail and a board. With each meeting we brought more building supplies. We hammered and sawed and painted. Before we knew it we'd built a friend*ship*. Together we've created quite a sturdy and beautiful vessel.

You have given me a great present—letting me know about your life with God. Our prayers together settle and center me. I learn about my faith because we are companions. You walk with me even when I can't walk. You don't even seem to notice I'm not up on my feet, treating me as if my illness is my challenge, not my identity. You encourage me to stretch and risk doing the impossible. You are the "yes" in my life.

Thank you for being my friend of the right hand. Thank you for not jumping ship even when my illness scares you. Your life brings me life. What more could you give a friend?

Love,
Barbra

CAT LESSONS

Journal
December 4, 1985

I'm in bed. Painful joints, feeling flimsy as my lace curtains. I can't be here. Not now. Christmas is coming with all it's preset demands. Like a time bomb. Ticking, ticking. And I can do nothing but rest while this needling wind blows. I'm in prison on this bed.

Curled like a princess in the middle of my quilts lies my cat, Prissy. I tried to move her off my feet. She flattened her black ears, flashed a peek from a blue slit eye and went back to sleep. Prissy needs her rest. After all she prowled around last night and hunted moths early this morning, She needs her rest so she can live her cat life. Nothing will redirect that need. I've never seen Prissy do a thing that wasn't good for her. In fact she does exactly what she wants, and I love her for it. Twitching tail, nervous whiskers and all. She has a great attitude about rest.

Maybe I could think of rest as accomplishing something. Supplying me with what I need. And I need rest like I need food and water. Rest is a good thing. Not a bad thing. While I lie here, I'll work on plans to simplify this Christmas.

Yes, I'll rest here with my cat and dream.

Barbra Goodyear Minar

MEDITATION

Journal
December 6, 1985

This resting business is serious. And I'm finding deep resting and resto-ration can come through meditation. When I shut my eyes and breathe and wait, I sense myself singing the ancient Psalms with my parents, grandparents, great grandparents:

Be strong, and let your heart take courage,
All you who hope in the Lord.[5]

Meditation reminds me that from birth to death, life is a holy thing. And celebration through sacred ritual with our Creator God is good.

We have a ritual to bless the children. Song and water and prayers: the sacred naming. The Baptism. We have a ritual to join lovers. Vows and rings and kisses: the sacred union. The Marriage. We have a ritual to have peace with God. The table and the bread and the wine: the sacred fellowship. The Communion.

After searching for Truth myself, I joined my people who, in Ro-man Catholic, Episcopal, Lutheran, Methodist, Congregational, Pres-byterian, and community churches through the centuries reached out for God and let Him embrace them.

We lay hands on the sick as healers. The hands and the prayer and the oil. We gather family and friends at the time of a death. Saying, "God the Father, Have mercy on your servant. May her soul and the souls of all the departed, through the mercy of God in Christ, rest in peace. Amen."

As Christians we prostrate, we kneel, we stand, we chant, we sway, we sing, we dance, we are silent. We have our great and holy rituals to honor the mystery of God. To be in communion with God.

Oh, God, I embrace you in the way of my ancestors. I embrace you as you meet me through your Spirit. I embrace you through Christ. I sit here listening for your voice not thundering in wind. Instead I hear, like the prophet Elijah, a quiet whisper speaking to my soul. I also must be still, and listen. Just as it has always been. Quiet me then, God. Through my meditation teach me to be still. And I shall be more whole.

GEORGIA:
THE BEST CHRISTMAS PRESENT EVER

December 27, 1985

Dear Frances,

I just had to let you know about this Christmas. Remember my vow of serving a large pizza and hot fudge sundaes? You know, "keep it simple, stupid!" Well, Gary's twin sister Marilyn phoned with plans to bring her family and Gram Dupuy up for Christmas day.

Still getting cytoxan pulses and spending a lot of time in bed, I was dragging around. My family was overjoyed they were coming, but, honey, I displayed the enthusiasm of a cat getting a bath. I *did* want to see them. I just couldn't figure out how to get the energy to pull it off.

Gary loves Christmas. Anyone who stopped believing in Santa hasn't seen Gary in holiday action. Near December 25th he's overcome with buying madness—especially bargains. Well, lucky for me he went into his usual shopping frenzy. He was terrific about grocery shopping, too. I began cooking one thing a day and freezing it, wondering when I pulled it all out what the Christmas menu would be.

The great feast day arrived. With Katherine's help I managed to get the table set, the food thawed and heated. I kept smiling and thinking, I'll call them to the table and I'll go find a motel. Just as we were sitting down, the doorbell rang. Standing on the front porch was my friend Georgia Weister dressed in black. I was about to ask her in for dinner when she tied on a white apron and put her finger to her lips.

"This is our secret. Don't say a word," she whispered. "Sit down. I'm serving dinner. Merry Christmas."

I stammered and hung onto the door knob. She turned me toward the dining room and gave me a gentle push.

"Sit down," she said with a low growl. I meekly slipped into my place. Everyone stopped talking and gawked as "the maid" deftly passed the roast beef to my mother-in-law.

"This is my friend and I . . ." Shaking her head, Georgia pulled her lips tight and scrunched her brow. My body melted into my chair. She passed the frozen fruit salad, poking me on the way to the kitchen. Then I got the giggles.

Without a question, everyone began eating and laughing and talking as if they'd been served Christmas dinner a million times by some stranger coming to the door.

Georgia Weister was the best Christmas present I ever had.

After everyone left I felt physically whipped but content. Resting under my down quilt this week, I've thought about the ups and downs of this year. I feel "weller"—on a path of more wholeness. Oh, honey, don't you remember when one pimple on our fifteen-year-old faces meant life was over. Now I know, not only to take my physical pulse, but my emotional and spiritual pulse as well.

I think living balanced in body, mind, and spirit is a triathlon event. Do you think we're up for that? It will take discipline every day of our lives. Remember when we were on the tennis team and grumbled about practicing backhands and forehands on the backboard. Over and over and over. Well, to be truly healthy we're going to have to exercise all we know! Over and over and over.

I think I've accepted that life is tough. Seems like Scott Peck agrees. I got his book for Christmas. *The Road Less Traveled*. He says:

> Once we truly know that life is difficult—once we truly
> understand and accept it—then life is no longer difficult.
> Because it has been accepted, the fact that life is difficult
> no longer matters.[6]

And, honey, that means we've taken a hammer to the happily-ever-after myth. We are not missing life if life ain't all easy and things gets a little windy! We are living proof life is tough! But tough or not, life is a fantastic experience. And full of God's surprises. I'm so glad I had Christmas dinner at my house!

New Year's blessings, my friend,

Barbra Kay

THE NEW CALENDAR

Journal
January 1, 1986

The New Year! I love the new calendar with its unmarked squares—clean spaces of life. Looking back through my old calendar, words, names, times, addresses are scribbled symbols of my everyday life. How fast I flipped those calendar sheets. My life sneaks by like a cat on a hunt secretly moving from morning to night. Padding softly. Stalking months on velvet paws until time's caught.

I become so frustrated with my unfilled hopes. It's in my soul that I should be jumping rope, dancing the tango, painting the kitchen, and planting tomatoes. Most of last year I spent trying to really deal with lupus. Learn more about it. Be more honest. Take responsibility for my life.

Last night I dreamed I was searching for a healthier body and came upon a woman strong and tan, muscled and energetic. I looked her over and said, "I don't have a strong body, but I have a strong spirit. Would you let me enter your body and become one with you?"

The woman agreed. I walked towards her, my thin, weak arms outstretched towards her powerful hands. Suddenly I froze, hugged myself like a treasure, turn and fled.

Oh, God, forgive me for not accepting myself—limitations and all. I never took clay and pressed out my form. I never demanded the Holy Mystery give me breath. I seem to be your idea.

When I feel weak, remind me of Your words in the Psalms that You are our refuge and strength. I want to have the exquisite experience of life. The suffering and the birth. The weeping and the laughing. Yes, the wind and the peace. I want to take it in and give it back to you, knowing, God of all seen and unseen, you embrace my fragile vessel with tenderness. You alone can stir all the life elements with wisdom and turn out gold. Oh Creator! Today I thank you for my life—all of it. Amen

Barbra Goodyear Minar

HIS EYE IS ON THE SPARROW

Journal
January 15, 1986

When I opened my stinging eyes this morning, they watered from light leaking through closed curtains. The sheets felt like sandpaper against my skin. My bones ached deep. When I took a sip of water, I felt sadness living in my throat—like a wad of bread that I couldn't swallow or cough out. I need to cry and melt it down. This new virus. Like a pebble that started a rock slide rumbling down a cliff, the first sneeze of this flu came on New Year's night. And the power of it poked a stick in the wolf's mouth. His anger makes red marks on my fingers. Claws a rash on my face. Drinks my energy.

Gary moved to Katherine's old room to avoid the flu, so I've been alone in my bedroom almost two weeks. Stale and musty, it smells like the big upstairs room where Grandmother Goodyear kept old lace dresses in tissue paper, and winter quilts and hat boxes and bisque dolls with sawdust-filled leather bodies in the oak trunk.

Tissue boxes, hot pad, wadded sheets, squashed pillows, stacks of unread books, the scattered <u>Los Angeles Times</u> share my bed. Water glasses, pill bottles, pens, my watch and rings crowd each other on my nightstand. Left over from Christmas my poinsettia drops yellow leaves by a heap of damp white towels. I wonder if I'll ever fold up my gray sweat pants and hang up the clothes mountain thrown over the wicker rocker? I wonder if I can ever pair up my shoes again and get them into my closet?

This morning when I tried to stand up, I squeezed my eyelids against the tears. Illness was eating another day of my new year. I walked to the kitchen on water legs with yesterday's tea cup . Like heavy dark spirits, sighs pushed themselves out of my chest as I surveyed the dishes in the sink, medical insurance papers on the table, spilled cat food on the floor.

I looked out the window at the deck. The birdfeeder. It was empty and swung back and forth. A determined black-headed English spar-

row darted around the empty cylinder. He sat on the silver rods making the long plastic tube swing. I slumped on my kitchen stool and watched him pecking at the seed hulls then flying away and coming back. He seemed desperate for food. Hungry for life. Just like me. A feisty fellow. Reminded me of Sir Winston Churchill. "Never give in. Never Never Never Never."

I pulled a sweater over my blue flannel pajamas, put on Gary's "Dallas Cowboys" baseball hat, pushed back the sliding glass door and stepped outside barefoot on the rough redwood deck. Winston Churchill instantly flew away, but I noticed him watching from the scrub oak. Raw morning air stung my face and cut into my lungs. Shivering, I buttoned the sweater at my neck and wished I had on slippers. I unhooked the feeder from its chain and pried opened the white plastic seed bucket. Plunging my hand into the yellow, black, and brown, I wiggled my fingers into comfort of the smooth seeds. I mixed them, scooped food into the feeder and hung it back up. Slipping inside I slide the door closed and sat at the window, rubbing my icy feet. I waited. In moments Churchill flew back and tucked his black head into the hole. Finding a feast, the sparrow ate as fast as he could, making chirp talk when he came up for air. Soon titmice, wrens, purple finches came from every direction chasing, fighting, gorging and squabbling! Going about their bird business, they got used to my face pressed close to the window, but scattered in shock when I started laughing.

I shoved my books over, climbed back into bed, nested in my pillow and laughed again, thinking of Sir Winston Churchill's persistence. I felt good rescuing him. And maybe he'd rescued me. I noticed the lump in my throat had melted.

"Never give in. Never Never Never Never."

SAYING YES TO LIFE

February 4, 1986

Dear Frances,

I saw this cartoon in the doctor's office. Hooked up to an IV a hospital patient is clutching her chest and staring in horror. A nurse is holding a giant iguana, shooting its tongue out over the bed. "Are you sure?" says the nurse. "Studies have shown that holding and caressing animals can dramatically speed a person's recovery!" Talk about heart failure! HA!

What's this I hear! You in a geology class at Gulf Coast JC. Good for you! Stop worrying about those field trips. When they come up, tell the instructor about your back and ask for help. In fact I think you and I both have to ask for more help, so we can say "yes" to life.

I don't know where we learned that it's cheating unless we do *everything* ourselves. Just remember when you delivered Connie. Honey you *screamed* for help and everyone came running. But when she was born you took all the credit.

Do you think it's pride that stops us from from reaching out? If that's true, pride could be keeping us from living a fuller life.

Last week Rebecca and Ann were planning a walk at Cachuma Lake Dam. As they talked, I sat wistfully listening, trying to be a good sport. Of course I couldn't go. I'd just started walking around the yard since my last flare. They'd be hiking in the sun. Probably for hours. Impossible. Then something rose up in me and I squeaked out, "I sure wish I could go." We tumbled the idea around and came up with a plan. We'd go late in the afternoon, ambling in the shady part. I could sit in the meadow when I got too tired while they hiked deeper in.

Oh, honey, that old gal Guilt. You know her—the gal with the rolling eyes, clucking tongue always yammering those "oughts and shoulds." Yeah, the one that spits "no-s" in our ear. Well, when I went to bed, Guilt rode in with me, claws dug in my shoulder and drove me crazy with her talk. "What if you caught cold and got sick again. What if you ruined their day . . ." You know. Finally I sat up and shouted, "Shut up. I'm going!" Gary rolled over and patted me. I think I scared him to death.

The next late afternoon we walked the short distance from Rebecca's home to the meadow's edge. Rebecca pushed down the top piece of barbed wire fence and Ann helped me over. I stepped into the deep wet grass, bending life under my boots and setting the pungent smell free. As we walked to a small creek through a patch of white violets and yellow sticky monkey flower, Rebecca pointed out bleached bones of a mountain lion's prey and a huge packrat's nest full of shiny tin and foil.

Winded and weak, I flopped in the grass and waved them on to explore the river and the dam. Sitting alone, I listened to frogs, birds, and mysterious rustlings. I lay on my stomach, looking at the world from the wildflowers' point of view. I dipped my hand in the creek and let the silky water eddy around my open fingers. I felt I was being touched by a lover and I shivered. I fished for small rock treasures and watched flashing silver minnows hiding close to the bank. Suddenly I sensed a presence. No sound. Just a change in space. A doe and two spotted fawns stood a few feet away—frozen except for the flick of an ear. A stone. I became a stone by the creek. In moments the doe walked toward me through the yellow buttercups and Indian paintbrush, leading her babies to the water. When she caught my scent, she startled and leaped away in slow motion. At safe distance she stopped with her babies and we stared at each other.

The girls returned, apologizing for leaving me so long bringing me a branch of bay leaves, a rabbit skull, three owl feathers, and stories of five blue herons.

Frances, what if I'd listened to Guilt? To think I almost didn't go! To think I would have missed my life by not risking. I know health is saying yes to all of life we can! Let's go for it girl!

Love,
Barbra Kay

BECOMING BREAD

Journal
March 20, 1986

The gift my young friend Jenny gave me this cold afternoon was more than the pink geranium in the wicker basket she set by my bed. It started simply enough. "I love the bread you made for Christmas. Would you give me the recipe?" When she stopped by Christmas eve afternoon, I'd just pulled two loaves out of the oven. She'd eaten a slab-lathered with butter and strawberry jam when the bread was really still too hot to cut.

I shook my head explaining I'm not much of a bread maker. Only make it for Christmas and Thanksgiving. If I can—if I feel good enough.

She looked away from me and picked at her bottom lip with chewed fingernails. Squirming a bit on the bed, Jenny cleared her throat. Then twirling a strand of auburn hair, she tucked it behind her ear. Touching her long arm, I pulled her hand into mine and waited until words began coming out in jerks, priming the pump of her gut. "A lot of symptoms. Tested for lupus. Came back positive. How to tell Mark? What about the wedding? What about children?" Talking in breathy phrases, she brushed tears away like unwanted gnats. "Could I—die? Why did God let this happen?"

Swimming through the sadness I felt for Jenny, I found my voice. Slow and calm. Waiting between questions. Stroking her shaking fingers. Looking into those wet amber eyes. Seeing that hunger. Feeling that fear. Knowing I could feed her truth and hope.

Wanting to shelter her from the wind, I pulled her close and rocked her like a small child. Holding her I realized she hadn't come for the recipe. Today she had come for bread. Like dough, I've been kneaded, and baked, then broken apart. And sometimes, like today with Jenny, a frightened starving soul stuffs my experience into her mouth and eats.

Jenny sat up, squeezed my hand and took in a long deep breath. She zipped up her yellow jacket and stood looking out my French doors.

"Thank you. Thanks," she said. And I walked her to the back door and watched her drive away.

Thank you, Jenny. It's a gift to be allowed to feed bread to His lamb.

Barbra Goodyear Minar

TOUCH: A GIFT FROM THE FINGERTIPS

Journal
May 19, 1986

Steven and Kathy's wedding's less than three weeks away. So today I had Mary cut my hair. Sighing, I sank back in the chair. My head ached, my joints hurt. Fatigue sucked at me like a giant leech. Mary said nothing but folded my collar, tucked a towel around my neck, and laid my head back in the sink. She hummed as she wet and soaped my head. Tenderly rubbing my scalp in gentle circles. Massaging my scalp and temples with her fingertips. Moving her thumbs against the back of my neck. Then smoothly wrapping my head in a warm white towel, she dabbed at the water dripping down from my hairline to my cheek as if she were wiping a rose petal. I sat still, hoping, she would never stop. Like a parched desert, my skin soaked up her touch all the way to my bones.

I closed my eyes as she brushed my hair with long slow strokes, lifted sections in her fingers and started to cut. She worked slowly around my head. Her closeness felt like a whisper. I noticed my headache was gone. My joints hurt less. A smile came into my body.

"Mary, I'm going to come here every day. You have healing hands." Mary turned the chair around and handed me a mirror to survey her work. "Everyone needs to be touched," she said. "Touch is part of what I do. You know Mrs. Baylor? Well, Mrs. Baylor's a regular. Comes ten o'clock every Saturday morning. It's a crying shame, but she tells me I'm the only one who touches her. I expect that's true. She being eighty-one, a widow and all. And Mrs. Baylor's not my only customer like that you know. That's why I love to go down to the Lutheran Home and do my ladies. Why, did you know Mabel Johnson's ninety-three? Has such back pain, but she never misses her appointment."

I know why.

Touch. I've been thinking about it all day. Everyone needs to be touched. Especially those of us with chronic illness. And often we're not—for lots of reasons, I guess. People are afraid to give us a hug. And we feel unattractive or unworthy, so sometimes we pull away. There's no fault here really, but I think the lack of touch makes me feel more distant, more separated from healthy life. I need to ask Gary to hold me. I need to hold him. I need to ask my friends for hugs. I need to give hugs away. I need to hold hands with someone. I need to stroke my cat down her back and let her rub against my legs. I need contact. I need touch, so I can connect with life.

God, I think I'll go visit Mrs. Baylor. She deserves to be touched more than once a week.

SURPRISE TORNADO

Journal
May 28, 1986

God, how quickly life changes. I thought Steven was calling me about wedding details. Instead his low voice lifted an octave when he told me. "Mom, I have cancer."

My firstborn. My son. He's supposed to be the bridegroom, filled with excitement of a sunrise. Instead, this! I would trade places with him in a breath. I've thought often of my death, but never his. It's as if I am on the front line. I should march into the unknown before him.

So I am here with him in Menlo Park, going to the cancer clinic at Stanford Hospital, fixing meals, unpacking boxes in his new honeymoon cottage, praying with him and praying in my closet. His anxious bride-to-be finishing nurses training in L.A. One day flung into another with only You, God, to sustain us. And how You have! We have eaten spiritual meat from the prayers of family, friends, and strangers. Somehow Steven and I have lived in the moment through the tests, consultations, surgery, tumor board, and the waiting by Your grace. Somehow we held back imagining the future.

Steven and I have talked until our eyes drooped, listened to jazz, laughed over family stories, and cried. The crisis has given us an unexpected gift of slowed-down space. Tonight we discussed what Billy Graham said about the human soul. He reminded us that the body, as precious as it is, will die. And often we care for our body but forget to care for our soul. "How foolish," he said. "How would we feel if the servant said, 'I've taken good care of the child's clothes but I've lost the child.'"

God, help Steven and me to use this experience to grow healthy, deep souls. I think about Abraham who gave you back his only son Isaac in total trust. I do the same. I release Steven and ask you for the gift of trust. For I am convinced, like Saint Paul, that nothing can separate our soul from Your love in Christ. Yes, God, not even death!

THE WEDDING DAY

June 7, 1986

Dear Steven,

Today is my forty-sixth birthday and your wedding day!

What an adventure we've had! Yesterday morning at the hospital was a trip! Finding out your CT scan looked great. The doctor doing a card trick and announcing your radiation can be put off until after your honeymoon. Everyone in the clinic clapping for the bridegroom. Then the powerful reminder of our gift of health when the young girl, rejecting her heart transplant, wished you joy.

Then to the Wine and Roses Country Inn where mother, father, sister, brother, grandma, cousins, aunts, and uncles stayed the night and you married your beautiful best friend this morning. Over two hundred guests witnessed your holy vows, applauded the kiss, drank a toast, tasted cake, danced the dance of celebration. Then you two were off, Oreo cookies stuck to the windows, tin cans rattling off the bumper.

Today I'm knitting memories of white silk with pearls and floating veil, blue satin dresses and black tuxedoes, gold rings and garden flowers, teary hugs and hearty handshakes. Be happy my son. Be filled with hope. Hope is the keystone of health in body and soul.

May God
keep you as two strong oaks
growing side by side
covering each other with your branches
giving each other strength by braiding your roots
making home in the shade of your love.

Blessings from your first best friend,
Mom

JAZZ MEDICINE

Journal
June 29, 1986

Drifting back from computer to bed these last weeks, I've been depressed. I resolve firmly in my mind I will not be depressed. But when Gary and I couldn't really celebrate our anniversary because of my stomach cramps and throbbing joints, I caught a foul wind that swirled my emotions. It usually helps when I list my blessings and practice gratefulness. But today depression is over me like a musty hooded cape, and the thick ties are tightly knotted at my throat.

    I had an idea. I dragged myself under this black cape to my music and found a jazz tape. I snapped it on and turned it up—loud. I stood by the speakers waiting for the vibrations. Notes came through my skin, caught a ride through my blood, and moved to the pumping of my heart. The flute untied the cords around my neck, the sax played a wild phrase that flung the cape through the wall. I tapped my feet as the bass talked sweet lows to me. I wanted to play a horn back. Oh, yes! Here it came again. Music flowing around my blood. I couldn't keep my body from swaying. For some people it may be Bach, Vivaldi, Mozart, Chuck Berry, or Elvis. But, baby, I love jazz. When everything in me feels dead, jazz brings me life!

THE GIFT OF FOCUS

July 2, 1986

Dear Carolyn,

Absolutely great news about Zondervan's interest in your book.
Good going, girl! Let me know the details!

Well, I have to tell you. Last week I got this letter in a white
envelope—my name typed on the outside. From *Virtue Magazine.*
It didn't look like a subscription request. I ripped it open whisper-
ing please, please. And YES! I'd sold my first article! I felt so crazy
happy I jumped on my bed. Only another writer could understand this nutty elation! It's a small piece on (of all things) the
difficulty of moving with tips to make it easier. Ha!

Oh, Carolyn, it feels good to publish. Sending writing into
the publishing world is like sending your baby into the street. You
don't know if she'll be run over by a truck or picked up and adored.
Most of my "babies" have been killed. It takes a lot of guts just to
keep sending them out. Don't you agree? Even with the fear I'm
think about a new book—a children's fantasy called *Lamper's
Meadow.*

I've been rolling this around lately—maybe a gift has come
out of my illness. You know I've always loved to tinker around and
never concentrated on any one thing. The shotgun approach to
life. Well, now I've had to "put down the shotgun and pick a target
and aim with a rife."

I've been reading *The Pursuit of Excellence* by Ted Engstrom.
He tells a joke about a guy who flits up to the ticket agent in the
airport and said, "Please, sell me a first class ticket." The agent
asked, "But where to, sir?" He answers "How could it matter? I got
business everywhere." Well, I had monkey business everywhere.
But without energy I had to focus, so I aimed at writing. However,
it's been scary with all work coming back in big self address enve-
lopes stamped "NO THANKS!" I've experienced a lot of failure,
but I like what Engstrom says. "Remember it's always too soon to

Barbra Goodyear Minar

quit. . . . Courage is the ability to 'hang in there' five minute longer."[7]

Thanks, Carolyn, for encouraging me all these months. I'm struggling with being balanced, not being compulsive, remembering the long process of learning. But today I take joy in this small beginning.

Cheers from a fellow scribe,
Barbra

PRACTICING PEACE

Journal
August 18, 1986

I told Dr. Gerber last week that my stomach's still rebelling. Everything's passing through with the force of a Yellowstone geyser.

"Get back on your banquet," he said.

Ugh! Since the mid-June, the BRAT diet. Bananas, Rice, Applesauce and Toast. I'd stayed pretty close to home—until Sunday.

Jeff called collect Saturday night from county jail. He got a DUI. My heart cramped, but I told Gary we couldn't bail him out. I scrubbed my eyes with my fists. We could go see him, I said.

So Sunday we drove to Santa Barbara. I'd never been to a jail before. Everyone stood in a stuffy, small room waiting—with children. A tiny newborn wrapped tightly in a thin, blue receiving blanket was going to see his daddy for the first time. A group of Hispanic women herded three young children who kept roaming outside and messing with sticks in a tiny pile of dirt. Their mother and father were both in jail. "The kids are living with me. I'm their madrina," explained a fortyish woman with a tattoo on her cheek.

From behind the bars the sheriff called visitors for each prisoner. We stepped on the elevator, pressed together, silently rode down in the tight metal box and stepped off into a windowless, cement block basement. Off to the right were narrow rows where glass partitions stood between prisoners and visitors with black phones connecting life to life. My stomach ached. There was no ventilation. I was sent down a row to station 77. Standing in the heat waiting for Jeff, I watched stories happening between the glass. The dark woman, eyes bruised with fatigue, unwrapped her infant and pressed him to the window. The father pushed his fingers on the glass, touching without touching and smiling. I waited. The woman beside me spoke strongly to her jet black son though the phone. "Read that letter I sent. Every line. Over and over 'til you memorize what I said. Do you hear me, Jacob?" He nodded his flat wide head up and down. I glanced at the mother. She at me.

"It's his first jail experience," she said. I nodded. He looked soft and young in front of his mother. He was crying and wiping his nose on his sleeve. "Good," said his mother. "You better cry!"

It was all rushing into me. The eyes, the tears, the dirty little children, the tired women. The heat. My face felt numb. I leaned against the glass. Rebecca's words circled in my mind. "Keep your skin on. Don't take in all the pain."

Jeff tapped on the window. His hazel eyes drooped at the corners. He looked clean. Teeth white. Funny how I noticed that. It was difficult to talk. His voice cracked over the phone. Sweat began running under my arms and between my breasts, drenching my shirt. Jeff said he borrowed another guy's toothbrush. I felt sick. He looked in my face. "I went to church," he said. "This morning."

"So did I," I said. "Your dad's here. He wants to see you." We put our hands together on the glass. When I pulled it away, my palm left a wet print.

"Pray for me, Mom." I nodded my head.

God, put your cloak over me and make me a prayer closet. Cover me from this wind and let me pray for these people. For Jeff. Then separate me from the pain. Put me back in my own body, so I can be healthy.

That night I rolled into a ball, and like a sad but comforting litany, I let my prayers rock me to sleep. God, fill me with your peace that covers the mountains. Fill me with your peace that covers the valley. Fill me with your peace that covers the sea. Fill me with your peace.

THE WOMAN AND THE JAR

Journal
September 21, 1986

Once there was a woman who sat by the gate of the world holding a jar in her lap. She sat and collected greed. She sat and collected beatings. She sat and collected lies. She sat and collected loneliness and poverty. She sat and collected hunger and cold. She sat and collected rape and murder. She sat and collected illness and death. As the jar filled up, the woman held it in her arms and her joints swelled, her head burned, her heart throbbed.

"Dear woman," said a Voice, "don't let that jar tip over into yourself. You'll die from the weight of the pain. Give it to Me." So the woman tipped the jar over—into the heart of God. And in thanksgiving she stood and danced in the sun.

Barbra Goodyear Minar

MESSIN' AROUND

Journal
September 23, 1986

Too much sadness. I needed a health break. While I was fixing my rice and bananas, my mind roved around like a hungry cat. Pawing around on the roof, walking the deck rail, running up the tree, stalking a phantom in the grass, pouncing under the porch. I wanted something. Something to make me laugh like crazy. Something like catnip.

Packing for college again, Katherine had suitcases open across her floor, mountains of dirty and clean clothes, books and tapes stacked on her dresser. I sat on her bed eating the last of my rice. "Hey, Kath, let's do something fun," I said. Katherine grinned and flung a pile of socks in the air. "All right!"

"First we gotta dress sort of—well funky," I said hoping right away she wouldn't wear her dinosaur slippers that make dinosaur mating calls when you stomp. We curled our hair and painted our nails bright pink. I put on a wild Hawaiian shirt with a button that said "Keep Your Chins Up." Katherine wore a red T-shirt that said, "Only God Can Tame A Woman," and off we went to Santa Barbara, me in a battered sun hat and Katherine in a bandana wrapped pony tail.

"First, let's get our faces done," said Katherine, driving into the mall parking lot. We walked though the warm afternoon wind through the glass doors of Robinson's. We slid onto tall stools at the cosmetic counter letting a young, straight-faced woman with alabaster skin and black hair twisted up and plunged with Chinese sticks powder and paint us. We tried to keep the giggles in our cheeks, but Katherine rolled her blue eyes one too many times, and I started laughing. "Sorry, sorry," I said to the wide-eyed woman, as Katherine fell off the stool and tears black with fancy new mascara ran down my cheeks.

Next we looked for a funny movie. <u>Peggy Sue Got Married</u> did the trick. While we rolled with laughter, I ate another banana and Katherine a big box of buttered popcorn. "Victory Women!" I shouted as *we drove back over the pass. "Go, Mom!" yelled Katherine, raising her pink fingernailed fist. "Victory Women!"*

Tonight I stomped around in Katherine's roaring dinosaur slippers. We took pictures and laughed until our ribs ached. Gary looked in on our insanity and went back to his paper. Tonight I was a happy tired when I crawled in bed. Katherine told me all her dreams, lying beside me while I rubbed her head the way I used to when she was very young. I'll miss her when she leaves next week.

Thank you, God, for catnip. Oh, thank you.

Barbra Goodyear Minar

IT'S ENOUGH TO SAY I MISS YOU

Journal
October 1, 1986

It happened again. Friday at El Rancho Market I saw Julie with her four-year-old Christy, feeling heads of lettuce. She glanced my way and then quickly pushed her cart down the aisle towards breads and cereals before I could say hello. I've known Julie a long time even before she put Christy in the preschool. I didn't have to be a brain surgeon to know she didn't want to run into me. But I like Julie, and Christy's a darling kid, so I just pushed my cart straight to breads and cereals, looked intently at the Fruit Loops and asked Christy which sugary cereal was she forbidden to eat. HA! Julie flushed red. "Oh, I didn't see you." She fumbled with the Grape Nuts while Christy yelled for Captain Crunch. "How are you? I've really meant to call or come by."

"I would have liked that," I said. "I've missed you. And Christy's grown so tall." I patted Christy's head. "Are you driving a car yet? You haven't gotten married have you?"

"NO! " Christy laughed. "I'm only a little kid. And I want Captain Crunch."

I felt like tossing a box in her mom's cart.

Julie looked at me from under her long bangs. "I guess I just didn't know what to say—about you being so sick." Her neck blotched and her cheeks blushed. "The preschool's not the same. I mean, I really miss you."

I squeezed her hand.

As Julie and I pushed our carts through the checkout stand, I felt her melt down. Her deep throated laugh punctuated her words as we exchanged simple stories. The next time I see Julie in the produce department, I bet we'll pick out lettuce together.

TAKING RISK

Journal
October 15, 1986

I didn't feel strong enough to travel when I bought my ticket, but I knew it was the right decision to make this long flight from California to Mississippi. I needed to come as much as Dad needed me to come. Back to the place I'd called home from age seven to twenty. Tonight in the tiny bathroom, bathing in the aged porcelain tub, I studied the gas heater I loved to light with long blue-tipped matches that warmed my thin body when I dressed for school in the winter; the toilet I threw up in after eating half a chocolate cake; the mirror that reflected the horrors of cutting my own hair when I was twelve; the room of discovering the first blood marking my womanhood. Part of the house has been remodeled, but the original windows in my old room are the same and the smells of the gardenia bush outside my window and bread from the big Colonial Bakery half a mile away are the same. I remember simple living. Both harsh and gentle scenes that made up my memory.

As I sat by my father's chair tonight I felt a sweet breeze. Holding his hand and laughing, tracing his blue eyes and full lips and lined face and silver hair with my seeing, I determined to exist in this moment of wholeness.

Barbra Goodyear Minar

PASSPORT TO THE HEART

Journal
October 30, 1986

I am twenty-three years younger than my father. Intelligent and healthy, vigorous and determined, he's led a life like a rushing river overcoming boulders and carving out the land. He never retired. Just changed directions. Winning prizes for his camellias, doing master woodworking in his shop, fishing the Gulf, rivers and bayous, singing in the church choir, cooking, traveling, reading and serving the community with his wife and friend Hazel. Now he's stopped. Put down flat. With nerve pain tearing from his knee up his back, sometimes he shakes and grinds his teeth. He can't concentrate on anything but the pain. The first surgery failed. The physical therapy made things worse. A new doctor has taken his case. Now pill bottles decorate the walnut chest he designed and built. Depression has swaddled him. Fear has become his keeper.

I have already visited this country. My illness issued me a passport. And even though we see it through different eyes, Dad lets me sit near him and be his guide. I can oil the hinge to open the door to his talk. I know how it feels to stop purposeful work and travel into an unknown frontier. He trusts me with his apprehension about seeing the new doctor tomorrow. We talk together about God. Sitting beside him is holy work.

The new doctor practiced her art. After tests, an injection and pain control, Dad is on his feet for short periods of time. He had a taste for crabs, so we all went to Shorties'. The strong reek of sea meat met us before we opened the wooden door. Not much stock but chewing tobacco, big cheap cigars, Rolaids, matches, Twinkies, Coke a Cola and all sizes of fresh Gulf shrimp, fish, and oysters on ice in a long glass case. The gray cement floor was wet from being hosed down.

"Got any crabs?" Dad asked the girl with the green frog earrings and matching necklace. "Just came in from Hugh's traps," she said with

MINA

a flat voice. "You like frogs?" I asked. "Not to eat," she said and she threw back her head, laughing at her joke. Dad laughed and Hazel laughed and I laughed, my eyes blurred with tears in this simple, wonderful moment without pain.

Barbra Goodyear Minar

STRENGTH IN COMMUNITY

Journal
November 6, 1986

I'm leading a small support group for moms from the preschool and community. While kids are in preschool and babies with sitters, we spend two hours just "being." Even though sometimes it's an effort to get there, it's a good break from my writing to see these young women on Thursdays—and a gift to find a place to give myself away.

This morning Marla sat with her arms crossed, red-eyed and silent. I introduced the idea that our unrealistic expectations color our attitudes. In fifteen minutes even the quiet women were exchanging insights and stories. Marla said she thought her husband was supposed to make her happy, and having a baby was supposed to make a couple closer. Looking down at the floor, she admitted that her colicky infant and worried husband brought on daydreams about her single days. When the group laughed in agreement, Marla was surprised.

Before closing, I shared the one thing I'm sure of. Each of us is totally known by God. He knows our deepest longings and cares about our lives even more than we do. Our parents, husbands, friends, and children can't love us as our Creator can. He loves us—completely.

There's an unspoken belief that if little girls are good, they'll be rewarded with a good life. When life is hard we think we're failing— failing to be good enough. Even with women's lib we still receive a subtle message that a woman's job is to make everyone happy. And then if we make everyone happy, someone will turn and make us happy.

What freedom to explore truth with these women! Life is hard. It's also glorious. And although we can gift husband, child, parent with our love, we are not responsible for their happiness. We are responsible for our own lives and emotions. Women can help women learn this in community. Women growing in health can travel together in a powerful way.

Although starting this group is a small offering, tonight I remember Marla's face as she examined ideas and talked with new friends. I think of her cooing over her wailing infant son and pulling the blanket back so I could see her treasure. "I liked being here today," she said softly. "I learned some things."

Oh, Marla, today you've given me purpose.

A NEW FRIEND

November 26, 1986

Dear Margy,
This is a thanksgiving note—for becoming my friend.

Remember the first time we met at Barbara and Mike's ranch party? As I recall I was feeling pasty and thin, sensitive about my ballooning face. I couldn't concentrate. When people were introduced their names flew out of my mind like birds. But I couldn't forget you. Black eyes sparking, you were laughing with another couple when Barbara introduced us. "I think you'll be good friends," she said. You were so powerfully beautiful, dressed in black with large silver hoops swinging from your ears and silver bracelets jingling as you said hello. We talked, then I moved away from all your light, never dreaming you and I could ever be friends.

Months later, arriving at an Arts Outreach board meeting, I sank in a chair and realized I was too sick to stay. You were there and as I got up, so did you. I have to leave, I said, feeling the heat on my face, trying not to cry. "You look like you need a hug," you said. And you hugged me big. I felt understood. I felt more whole.

One morning I broke from my writing and went to the mailbox to find one of the most precious requests of my life.

A Card. Saying. You. Wanted. Me. To Be. Your Friend.

How could a woman with the vital life of a red tailed hawk be interested in a relationship with a slow box turtle? Of course, I said YES! And since that day we've said "yes" to each other a thousand more times. It's difficult enough for dear old friends to brave my illness with me. But you walked right into the wind with me and we started a new friendship.

Your reach toward me, starting with that hug, says there's something very interesting to a hawk; something very valuable about a box turtle.

There's no doubt about it, Margy. Your love over coffee and lunch, picnics and poetry, books and prayers, birthdays and funerals, sharing and silence brings me healing. Yes, there's no doubt about it!

Fondly,
Barbra

Barbra Goodyear Minar

CHANGES

I tried to ignore the hints and rumors. But now it's reality. Gary's been transferred. Just came home from work, put his briefcase on the table and said it. Transferred.

The wind whipped at me. My face went numb.

"Not until January." Gary's voice broke through my daze. "Work's closing down here. I'm lucky to get a job, and Long Beach is only three hours from Solvang. Long Beach is a great city. It'll be an easy move."

Easy move. Oh, God. Three hours or three thousand miles. Packing boxes. Selling the house. Leaving friends, my church. Leaving Dr. Gerber. I know the routine. We've moved five times. I know the price.

"What do you think," he said getting a Pepsi out of the refrigerator. What do I think? How can I think? My brain's turned to runny oatmeal. Transferred. Just like that. My life put through the paper shredder. Start over. My head thumped deep inside. Fatigue drained the blood from the soles of my feet and my spirit floated away from my body.

Gary talked on and on. Excited. Enthusiastic. Encouraging me. Finally, I gathered myself back inside my borders. I thought of packing dishes. My hands pulsed and throbbed red. Some nights I can't even set the table. What did I think? he asked again.

I think I wish I had a broken leg, an amputated foot, a bleeding wound on my cheek so he had visible clues about lupus. This hidden wolf that lives uninvited in the caves of my body. If only Gary could see his narrow eyes, his tail, his horrific teeth. If he only knew how much work it is to keep him sleeping. I want to live. The best life I can.

Gary looked at me, waiting. And finally my words came out. Words mixed with tears, but words so brave I was astounded. "I'm not sure," I said, "that I can make a move." My chest swelled and collapsed. The words shot like arrows and hit the bull's-eye. My heart knows. My body knows. My soul knows I can't make a move.

Gary shook his head, then left for the den and flipped on the TV. I put my head down on the kitchen table and let tears wet the place mat. Maybe this was the ultimate pressure that would smash us to pieces. Maybe I'd gone too far. Still I can't move. God, I know I'm not responsible for having lupus, but I am responsible for making good choices for my life. Guide me in the ways of love for Gary—Guide me in the ways of love for myself.

Barbra Goodyear Minar

TAKING RESPONSIBILITY

Journal
December 2, 1986

*The decision about the move is made, but even after knowing my truth,
I wrestled like Jacob with the angel in dreams and day visions asking
for confirmation. I'd see Gary leaving without a kiss, without a touch.
He'd push out the screened door. Face dark, shoulders bent, he'd climb
into his brown Datsun, suitcases and boxes crammed to the ceiling in
the back seat. Looking behind him, he'd back out of the driveway. Never
waving goodbye. Hoping to see the lift of his hand, I'd wait until he
was out of sight. Then I'd cover my face with my hands.*

*Some days I felt stronger. Maybe I could do it. I'd daydream the
moving van into the drive. Packers carrying out boxes of bubble-wrapped
blue calico china again. Gary and I signing escrow papers for a quaint
little house with a red tile roof in Long Beach. Gary would hold me.
Ready to celebrate. Then my resolve would melt like cotton candy in my
mouth and I'd feel angry. Going or staying, I betray myself.*

*It was good to pray for wisdom. To work on a solution with Gary;
to talk with Ann and Rebecca and my children; to grapple with it in
counseling; to take in Dr Gerber's gentle counsel. Moving would bring
great stress. Stress is my major enemy. So risk my decision. Don't move
with my husband.*

*The decision needs compromise. It holds both good and bad parts,
but we can try it. Gary will commute during the week, coming home on
weekends. I will join him some weeks. Our friend Francie will rent a
room from us. She'll give me a hand when I need it. But I feel afraid. A
wife should go with her husband.*

*Sometimes I really long to know the future but this anonymous
parable Carolyn sent me speaks the truth.*

*And I said to the man who stood at the gate of the year: Give me a
Light that I may tread safely into the unknown! And he replied: Go out*

into the darkness and put thine hand into the hand of God. That shall be to thee better than light and safer than a known way.

God, take my hand.

Barbra Goodyear Minar

CLIMBING NEW HILLS

January 3, 1987

Dear Frances,

Honey, this is your New Year's (see the little balloons?), Valentine (see the little hearts?), and Washington's birthday (see the little hatchets?) card. I'm trying to economize my energy. HA!

Well, I survived another holiday season! Sort of. We had an "on the road" season—Christmas both here and in Northern California so we could see all the kids. The best thing I did was sing. It's been a long time. Since high school. Remember us yawning first period in the alto section under poor Miss James? Well, our church choir invited others to practice with them for a concert. I didn't know if I could stand up that long, much less oil my rusty voice and sing. But I tried. AND I DID IT! I grinned through the whole performance. Boy, were my knees shaking when we sat down. Now I'm flat for awhile. But it was absolutely worth risking something new!

I'm certain my activity level bouncing up and down confuses my family and friends. Last week I met my friend Joan in the bank parking lot. I was almost embarrassed to see her. She's asked us over for dinner a hundred times, and I've never had the energy to repay her. So I told her I felt bad about it. She laughed and said, "Forget it. Who's keeping score?" Yesterday she brought me a small box. I read the card.

"Beleek china is from Ireland. My Aunt Nita had one cup and saucer, and it always fascinated me because of its fragile beauty. Once as I was praying for you, God let me see that you're like a piece of Beleek. A fragile vessel and yet strong because you allow Jesus to be your strength. I knew someday I wanted to give you a piece of Beleek, so here it is. A little way to express a very large love."

I took the lid off the box and lifted the white porcelain heart to the light. Oh, yes, Frances, we're fragile. But when we're weak, God can be strong through us.

Maybe we can't climb mountains, but let's pick a couple of new hills this year and give 'em a try.

Love,
Barbra Kay

CHANGE: THE CONSTANT IN LIFE

Journal
March 28, 1987

The only constant in life is that things change. Just when we steadied ourselves in the Valley for another year of dry hot winds and drought, looking at the burned hills from summer that never sprouted green from needed winter rains, just when we sighed over the low water in Cachuma Lake, just when the cattlemen sold their cattle for lack of grazing land, just when we adjusted to the lack of water in the creeks, not watering our lawns or washing our cars, it rained. And rained and rained.

Change after twenty-six years. All my children are gone. I have no job. Gary moved out. Francie moved in. I'm living in between two homes. How can I deal with all the unknowns? My bed empty during the week. My nights lonely but free. I step out calling to the Spirit to take me into these places I've never been before.

Just this week I read again Madeleine L'Engle's <u>Walking on Water</u>. She remembers Isaiah with all his flaws saying like a courageous, inno-cent child to God, "Here I am send me." Isaiah understood God's Spirit would be with us, freeing us from earthly restrictions. He writes

> *'When you pass through deep water, I am with you; when you*
> *pass through rivers they will not sweep you away; walk*
> *through fire and you will not be scorched, through flames and*
> *they will not burn you.'*

> *"I clung to those words," Madeleine says. "I know there will*
> *be days alone with flames. I too anticipate flames. But when*
> *a fire rushes through there's room for new growth."[8]*

Not everyone understands. I had a feeling I was in for a test when Rosalie approached me outside the church, holding the crown of her black felt hat to keep it from blowing off. "Well, do you mean it? 'You didn't move with your husband.' My Larry would never stand for that!" Her eyes pinched together under her frown, as I awkwardly defended my situations, mumbling that had we decided
. . . for the sake of my health.

"Well, I know plenty of fine doctors in Long Beach. It's a big city." She adjusted her hat and patted my sleeve. "I wouldn't let my husband go by himself. Especially these days." She arched her penciled eyebrows. "I believe those words 'whither thou goest I will go,' but I'm sure you know best."

Know best? I felt water washing over my feet, hearing Rosalie's echo. How do I know this is the absolute right thing? Now the water was up to my waist and, as I resurrected my doubts about us living apart, water closed over my head. I bobbed up and down all evening trying to keep from drowning.

As Gary packed his suits and ties, I rolled his clean socks. "Make sure you get the check to the bank in the morning," he said, not looking up.

"Want to take some of that casserole for tomorrow night?" I asked, smoothing a stack of undershirts. "No, save it for yourself. I have my own routine. Just swing down to the Naval Base and pick up food." I grabbed his hand and felt the edge of his gold band. He pulled me into his arms on the bed. We lay there breathing together. He lifted his head to read the clock. "Gotta go. It's either now or four in the morning." I followed him out to the car. He loaded up, backed down the driveway and then stopped and blinked his lights goodbye. We both are walking on water.

THE DOCTOR'S PRESCRIPTION

Journal
April 15, 1987

This morning Dr. Gerber felt the bluish ulcers on my toes, listened to my chest, and looked over the lab work as I sat on the end of the paper-covered table in his office. I feel bad, I said. "Where?" Dr. Gerber lifted his chin, his light blue eyes intense. "Your stomach? It's pretty tender. I think we need to up your steroids." I bit the inside of my cheeks, demanding the water in my eyes go back to the sea. "I feel guilty," I said, "I feel bad about being separated from Gary. Having him live alone."

Clearing his throat Dr. Gerber took my hand. "You have a lot of compassion for everyone—but yourself. If a friend of yours had vasculitis and couldn't eat because of stomach pain, I bet you'd really care. You'd be kind. Barbra, you feel guilty about having lupus. It's not your fault, but how you deal with it is your responsibility. Not moving was a responsible choice. Now here's my prescription." He whipped out his prescription pad, wrote something down, and put it in my hand.

Barbra Minar—
Must do something kind
for herself
3X per day.
Taking the pad back, he added,
For the rest of her life.

DRESSING UP THE BONES

April 20, 1987

Dear Katherine,

Fun talking with you on the phone last night and laughing about our nutty movie adventure last September! Let's plan another crazy day when you come home.

I promised you I'd keep you informed about my body. Well, it seems I need to increase my medication because I'm having a flare right now. Last week Glendora Gloom looked back at me everytime I glanced in the mirror at my round, blotchy face. So I decided to do something about her. First I polished my toenails blue. Don't laugh! Really I did! And if you'd left the dinosaur slippers, I'd have those on.

Seriously, I need to pay attention to how I look so I've started putting on makeup every day and wearing purple. I found some makeup that covers the rash popping up on my cheeks. I even got Ann to drive me to the beauty shop so I could get my hair cut. It's amazing how much healthier I feel.

Really, Katherine, maybe being tender with myself is like singing a love song all the way to my bones. Sometimes when I'm sick, I feel angry at my body for letting me down. I want to leave my skin home and live somewhere else. But being compassionate with myself, telling my body it's a flaming hero, has turned my thinking around. After all, it's gone through many wars and keeps recovering from the battle wounds. Come to think of it, I have a pretty fantastic body. And it deserves some dollin' up.

When you come home will you pluck my eyebrows? They're out of control and I need to look *beautiful!*

Love you,
Mom

P.S. Fantastic news! Steve's medical reports came back clean as a whistle. No cancer!!

NAPS

Journal
April 29, 1987

I know I'm supposed to get plenty of rest. I know naps are like pieces of gold that can buy you more energy for the rest of the day. But sometimes I shoot off like a sparkler, ignore the exhausting wind blowing into my face, and just drag my body along.

Yesterday I shopped through El Rancho Market picking up granny smith apples, vanilla yogurt, bagels and cream cheese, a chicken and big Idaho baking potatoes because Katherine was coming home. I stopped by the post office and mailed off Hazel's birthday gift. Went by the bank to deposit a check. By the time I unloaded the groceries I felt like a swing with my ropes cut. And I still wanted to make up Katherine's bed. How could I get the bottom sheet on with that fourth corner you have to yank into place? How could I manage to pull up the heavy blankets and bedspread? How could I stuff the pillows into the pillow cases? As I struggled with the bedding, my heart raced and I began to cough. I still had all the medical insurance to process. I wanted everything finished, so Katherine and I could spend time together. At least that was my rationale for pushing myself. But the thought of sitting down with all the paperwork made my eyes heavy.

Just then the cat jumped into the middle of the down comforter I'd just smoothed. Her eyes slices of blue, Prissy circled around making a nest. Lying down she purred a little purr and went to sleep. Just like that! Took a nap! In the middle of the day! With all the work to do! I stood over her with my hands on my hips. She smiled and flicked her whiskers, dreaming a cat dream.

I was about to scoop her off the bed. But I took another look at her relaxed body and easy breathing. Prissy was smarter than I was. She was taking a nap when she needed one. Yes! Right in the middle of the day. Maybe I could lie down just for a second. Just to rest my eyes. Only for a moment. I slipped off my tennis shoes, lifted up the comforter and slipped between the fresh sheets, letting the mattress hold my weary body.

I began to float. When I woke, Prissy was stretching her paws beside me.

I was feeling her soft fur and rubbing her stomach just as Katherine swung her green duffel bag through the door. "Oh, Mom, how wonderful." She kicked off her shoes, grabbed Prissy and climbed under the covers. "Traffic was awful. I'm beat. Could we take a little nap?" I thought it was ridiculous to go back to sleep, but Prissy settled down and shut her eyes. And I wanted to be at least as smart as my cat. So I rolled over.

A nap is a healthy gift to give someone—especially yourself.

THE LISTENING TABLE

Journal
May 2, 1987

*Yesterday Linda came to visit. A mutual friend thought I could help her.
She sat at my kitchen table like a sad child while I made lemon tea. I'd
only met Linda once before at a baby shower. I remembered her young
and tan, standing in the middle of the room talking with dancing
hands about her hopes to hike in Switzerland. Now her thin face was
white as the paper napkin she pleated by her cup. After pouring the
steaming water over the tea bags, I sat down. She tapped her fingers
lightly on the table, saying she felt silly about being with me. She didn't
really know what to say. Her soft voice faded into the walls. She stared
out the window.*

*I touched her nervous fingers and felt the trembling. I wanted to
tell her all sorts of things. Things about dealing with losses, living with
her illness, finding support. But something held me back.*

*"You don't have to talk," I said. We sat in silence sipping our tea.
Little by little her words trickled out. "How could—how could I—have
multiple sclerosis? I was jogging one Saturday and on Sunday one side
of my body didn't work." I poured another cup of tea. Finding her voice,
she locked her pale eyes on mine. The press of the river broke the log
jam. She talked. It was all there: the grief, the fear, the anger, the
loneliness. Our stories all have the same themes, but Linda's, like everyone else's, was incredibly unique.*

*"I got so many things I want to do. So many plans. And how am
I going to keep working? I mean, I gotta hold on to my medical insurance. I gotta raise my two kids. My two kids." She held her face in her
hands. She told me about her divorce. How maybe it was a mistake, but
she couldn't do anything about David now. Now that she had MS.
Everything was too complicated.*

*As afternoon shadows fell across the kitchen, her river slowed down.
Linda put her cup in the sink. "Oh, sorry I stayed so long. I mean, I
didn't want to tire you out."*

I asked if I could hug her. Fitting under my chin, she stood for some moments, letting me put mother-arms around her small back. "I'm honored to hear your story. Linda, you're honest and brave." I squeezed her.

"Yes." She looked up and tilted her head. "I'm deciding to be brave." I swear light came out of her face.

MAKING HOME WHERE YOU ARE

Journal
May 4, 1987

I've come with Gary to Long Beach this week. After he goes to work, I write here in the hotel at a little round table with two wooden chairs. A large TV sits like a big eye on the long dresser. Heavy green black-out drapes pull across the window. Two queen size beds fill up the room, leaving only a narrow path to get to bath or door. A huge mirror hangs flat on the wall. When I pass by, I'm shocked by the middle-aged woman with the pale face who follows my stare.

Today I got up early and had a long time of prayer. Then I went to my computer and worked on <u>Lamper's Meadow</u>, but by mid-morning I felt like I was choking in a cell.

Unbolting the brass lock, I stepped outside. It was hot. Too hot for April and thick smog lay overhead like a gray shroud. I felt good about being here for Gary, but I ached for home and the valley. Steady rains have come since February. Shoving up from their winter graves, plants are exploding from their seed cases. The great oak groves spring green overnight. Cows are dropping their calves in the pastures. Deer are hiding their fawns in new grasses. Creeks are finally flushing with water. Folks are riding rubber rafts down the Santa Ynez River as it flows through our town to the Pacific. If I were stronger I could drive myself home.

As I stood in the hotel courtyard under the weight of the city noise, I noticed the flit of a tiny bird. A hummingbird. Zipping by me, she flashed iridescent blue, green, and magenta. She flew by again. This time I kept my eye on her as she dove to a newly planted tree. Hanging on a tiny branch was a gray-brown nest no bigger than my thumb with an orange thread running through it. The mother sat in her nest, head poking up to protect her eggs. She looked so pitiful, really. Nest clinging to a branch the width of a pencil. Her home was naked, unprotected. Hanging at human eye level. But there she was. Faithfully guarding her family-to-be. Confident she could build a home no matter where she lived. I shall name her Grace.

I went inside and plumped the bed pillows and taped pictures of the kids to the mirror and called my husband to wish him a good morning.

ANNIVERSARY WONDERINGS

June 28, 1987

Dear Gary,

It's 10:45 p.m. and I can't sleep. After being apart, our weekend's been filled with being together. And we gave each other the best of ourselves. When you drove away tonight I was flooded with things I didn't say. Even after twenty-seven years of knowing you, I still feel shy sometimes—tongue-tied like I felt at fourteen. Long-legged and awkward. I'm wondering what you're thinking on the long drive back to the city. I'm wondering if you're thinking about us or setting your mind free, listening to Johnny Cash sing about "the hurtin' life."

Your slippers are still by your side of the bed. I can put my fingers into the dent you left in your pillow this morning. I feel lonely for you and at the same time looked forward to what my single life will teach me tomorrow.

As you come and go, as I stay, I'm realizing I'm growing—in ways I hadn't figured on. I'm doing some growing up in this protected space, meeting myself every morning and deciding what I need to do to grow healthier in body, mind, and spirit. I can't blame my lack of discipline on your needs. I can't take out my fear or frustration on you. I can't hide behind your shirt. I'm face to face with me.

Not moving to Long Beach was one of the hardest decisions I ever made. Thank you for helping us stay rooted here. Thank you for committing to our "us" in this new arrangement. I'm nurtured here surrounded by old committed friends, our church, my doctor, my writing. And you coming home every Friday night. With all this support I'm learning to walk into the wind.

Love,
Barbra

P.S. I think I can finish *Lamper's Meadow* this week. What an incredible feeling to end a book!

Barbra Goodyear Minar

DANCING

Journal
July 8, 1987

The flight to Mississippi was challenging, and it's very hot. So I'm taking lots of naps, going to bed early, and trying to sleep late. Perhaps the hours in the room of my youth is causing the many dreams.

Last night I dreamed I wanted to dance. I walked into a huge auditorium for an audition. Waiting for my name to be called, I kept smoothing my long flowing skirt and checking the white ribbons on my toe shoes. The music played. I was called out and went spinning onto the stage, the blue of my skirt floating around my body. Suddenly I was winded. I tried to keep dancing, but my legs wouldn't hold me up. I pushed hard but stumbled, my toe shoes clacking against the wooden floor. I fell, tangled in my skirt. The music faded and the man with a clipboard said, "Sorry. Good potential but no stamina."

I woke up crying and lay in my bed, trying to make sense out of the dream. I remembered taking ballet as a ten-year-old at Miss Evonne's Dance Studio on second street. I pedaled my bike from school to class, but by the time I arrived I was often too tired to dance. Miss Evonne said resting wasn't acceptable. My mother explained that I'd had rheumatic fever when I was younger. Miss Evonne clapped her hands for us to line up in position one. "If she comes to my class she must dance," said Miss Evonne. I quit taking lessons, but I remember going to the Gulfport High School Auditorium that spring and seeing my friends dancing in pink ballet tutus and tights with flower wreaths on their heads. I cried.

I should be able to dance. I've twirled around with scarves as long as I can remember. I've always carried dancing in my heart. And a feeling that I am inferior because I can't force myself to "get up and dance." It's time to heal—to put that dream to rest. And the physical activities dancing symbolize. Swimming at the ocean with my family, playing tennis with friends, kayaking with Gary, backpacking alone up a mountain trail. High energy is like the power of floodlights, but there's also a valuable place for the energy of candlelight.

Perhaps health is seeing things in a new way. Why, I can dance. I can dance—with my eyes, with my words, with my prayers. And sometimes even on my feet.

Barbra Goodyear Minar

A MATTER OF SEEING

Journal
September 9, 1987

Indian summer. The thermometer read 97 degrees in the shade twice this week. Frightening hot afternoon winds are blowing, threating us with high fire conditions. When I stepped outside yesterday to get the paper I took a look at my yard. My yard is hideous. Burned up. Trees need pruning. Flower beds need compost and new bedding plants. Roses need feeding and the dead blooms cut off. How can weeds grow green and tall while the shasta daisies turn brown and droop? I can't even find the red stepping stones leading off the porch, they're so covered with dandelions. Everything needs watering, but part of the irrigation system is clogged up with earwigs and gravel so the lawn has brown swirls where the water fails to spray. Brown pine needles blanket the junipers, and the honeysuckle is climbing across the bedroom window. Gophers make mounds all over the yard, as if they're having a family reunion. It's all hideous.

After dinner I sat in the middle of my garden on my blue kneeling pad looking for the silver lamb's ear Ann gave me from her farm. With my rusty spade I worked the ground around the choking soft leaves. I remember putting lamb's ear carefully in the garden following Ann's instructions and now it's dying. I pulled up grass and dandelions and tall wild oats, making a pile on the lawn. Suddenly I felt my hand and arm tingling. Red ants! I jumped up, pulled my longsleeve shirt off and brushed madly. Finally cleaned off, I flopped on the deck exhausted. My head ached, my joints hurt. And I had accomplished nothing but making a small pile of weeds I was too weak to haul away.

Last night, my body pulsing with pain, I thought about the yard. It's just too much, and I can't do the work, but I can't stand the mess. If I didn't have this darn lupus I could roll up my sleeves and clean up the place. I fell asleep on my hot pad, dreaming of weeds growing up over the windows.

Today Maria came by from the trailer park in Los Alamos. Rubbing one puffy red hand over the other, she talked about her need for a specialist to help her with her rheumatoid arthritis. "When Jerry's company changed insurance policies, we didn't realize I couldn't go to my doctor anymore." She sipped her tea. "Gosh, I'm just not sure what to do next. The doctor I'm assigned to is nice enough, but she doesn't know much about RA."

Looking into Maria's anxious eyes as she talked, I felt my stomach knot. "Losing Dr. Gerber would frighten me," I said. "Really frighten me! I can't believe you're so cheerful." "Something will work out if I keep trying," she said. "And, gosh, anyway today's a good day. I'm here with you in all this beautiful yard." She opened the French door and let a blast of heat in the house. "Just look at your flowers! And all that space."

I waved my hands telling her the yard was a total mess. Gary's gone all week and I didn't feel up to working out there. "Course you don't! Just have to think of things in a different way. Like you don't have a formal garden. You have a country yard, and I think country yards are supposed to be kinda messy. Makes them more friendly." She limped onto the deck and pointed to our ancient oak tree. "Think of having that old beauty living in your own yard. Gosh, I love it."

I put on my sun hat and dug up some lamb's ear and snapped off starts of red geranium for the pots on Maria's porch. Tonight a soothing breeze brought me sweet smells of summer as I sat on the deck eating my salad. And I lifted my eyes from the weeds and watched the half-moon rise through the branches of the oak tree that shine over my country yard.

Barbra Goodyear Minar

STRESS BUSTERS

January 2, 1988

Dear Frances,

Oh, honey, I hear you. Holidays are great but STRESSFUL. And we pay a price. I hate to admit that my body's so affected by stress. But it seems every January I'm writing to tell you I'm sick. All the literature on diseases marks stress as an enemy. It would be hard enough if living stress-free meant trying to avoid bad things like working on taxes or having a mean uncle staying in your house for six months. But no—we have stress with *good* things like buying a new home, getting a new job, going on a great trip, having people over for dinner.

Remember the emotional-physical chart we started keeping years ago? Well, I still keep mine up. And there really is a connection between stress my physical problems.

Frances, what if we write each other a bunch of stress busters. Just write anything that would help no matter how crazy it sounds. Okay, I'll start.

- Bank and shop by mail whenever you can.
- Get rid of anything that doesn't work right, like old alarm clocks that don't keep time or radios that buzz, or mystery keys that don't open anything.
- Simplify your life. Dig through your closets and get rid of old clothes. Empty the kitchen of appliances you don't use.
- Exercise. Walk wherever you can.
- Reward yourself after you've done something difficult. Call a friend. Take a nap. Watch a video. Read a book. Take a bubble bath.
- Talk about it. If emotions are boiling, stress is building up like steam in a teapot.
- Create fun in your life. Go to the movies, talk to a child on the phone, make up jokes.
- Pet your cat.

- Keep emergency supplies of basic needs like extra medicine, soaps, toothpaste, toilet paper, and use them only in an emergency.
- Start early. Allow extra time to arrive for appointments so you don't feel rushed(this really helps me!).
- Be prepared to wait. Bring along a book or letters to write in the doctor's office.
- Make a special place of your own. I have a rocker in a corner of my room with a purple afghan my friend Lindy made me and a pile of books.
- Relax your standards. Remember a perfectionist is suffering from a mental disease, and I don't need another disease!
- Laugh every day (I never miss the funnies).
- Practice gratefulness every day.
- Pray every day.

Okay, honey, see if you can beat that!

Love ya,
Barbra Kay

P.S. Oh, yeah, I forgot my all-time favorite. Eat a hot fudge sundae for lunch.

CHOOSING

Journal
January 2, 1988

The thing I can't write to Frances is the thing I can hardly write here. Jeff didn't come home for Christmas. Just passed through with his friend Vicky to have a meal and pick up his gifts. He stooped like an old man, his sad smile disappearing under his mustache. He looked sick. I felt desperate about him. And the desperation sat on my chest like a collapsed stone wall. I needed help.

I called my Al Anon sponsor, Barbara. Barbara was raw with me and honest. She shared the story of the loss of her infant granddaughter, telling me that no matter what we do, we can't stop the coming of another's death. The best we can do is to live fully and grow up ourselves—learning about the ways of Joy until our bodies dissolve and our spirits escape to the One who made us. Barbara leaned near me. "Jeff has been dealt a tragic genetic blow," she paused and held her fingers against her graying temples, "which it appears he will die from. God may intervene, but there's nothing you can do to interrupt the chemistry or change the flow of his life." She gently pressed my hand. "But you have a choice. Live your life to the fullest."

Again, I have to practice letting go and living my own life.

What a strange thing it is to have a child. I feel so responsible for his outcome. It's absolutely true I was a vessel for birth and human care, but the deeper reality is that from the moment of conception he was out of my control. The act of energy in lovemaking, the act of energy during conception was my way of participating with my Creator. My unborn took his form separate from the two lovers—yes, even separate inside me in his own water world. Shaping, growing into an original creation. When his time was full, he broke completely free of my womb—and yet was completely helpless, needing hands and breasts and love. Still, the baby was far more separate than I knew. We, mother and child, were not one. We were always two. And the moment of his first breath, he began his journey toward his last breath. There is nothing I could ever do to change the destiny of dust to dust. Yes, I needed to let go from the beginning.

Today I'm deciding to live healthy. I'm choosing to be grateful for my husband, Katherine, Steven. And grateful for Jeff and the lessons I'm learning about life through him.

WISDOM IN A CHILD

Journal
February 17, 1988

I slipped my manuscript into a folder and drove to the Meeks to read two more chapters of <u>Lamper's Meadow</u> to Christin. Whenever I think about her battle with liver cancer a windstorm starts in my stomach, and when I pray, the windstorm turns into a hurricane. With all my being I don't want her to have cancer. It's one thing for me to battle with illness. I've had a full life already. But Christin's only fourteen! It's not fair!

Christin was about seven when her mother, Barbara, had Ann home school her. The first time I met Christin at Ann's farm, I was captivated. "Do you believe in angels?" she asked, illuminated blue eyes searching my face. "You should you know." Yes, Christin possessed the rare quality of a pure child with a wise old soul.

Now Christin has lost her long blond hair. She looked as thin and white as baking powder. Dark half moons sweep under her eyes. But those clear eyes. They penetrated my core. While I read, she curled up on the couch in a oversized sweat shirt. "Good," she said when I finished. "Good. Except the part about Mrs. Mole talking to King Lamper about the kids. Who is she exactly? Their teacher? Better make it more clear." Without a pause she jumped into the questions feet first. "You've been sick a long time?" "Yes," I answered. "And were you mad?" I told her I was too sick to be mad in the beginning. But, yes, I got mad. Christin sat up, leaned forward and squinted at me like a lawyer. "God loves me, so why's He letting this bad thing happen?"

I stared at Christin and stammered out, "I don't know." Christin laced her long thin fingers across her bald head. "Well, what do you think?"

I told her I believe if I put the bad things of my life into God's hands and let Him have control, because He loves me, He will teach me and deepen me and heal me in different ways.

"Jesus is going to heal me," stated Christin. She smiled suddenly, her face radiant. "And I'm going to tell others all about Him."

Christin asked me when I could come again and read. I'll listen to her questions, too, but I feel that hurricane. Oh, God, do heal Christin! Help me trust you with her life!

THE DEEPEST HEALING

July 12, 1988

Dear Frances,

Oh, honey, I love to get your letters, but your questions! Now that's another story. But since today's your birthday, I'll give it my best shot.

Okay. Does God heal people when they pray? I pray for Jeff to be healed from his addiction every day, and even though he's still sick, I know Janice, Dick, and Charlie who are recovering. I've read accounts of physical healings even in the *Reader's Digest*. When we lived in Ohio, I knew a six-year-old girl with an inoperable brain tumor. She was healed through prayer. Right now I'm praying (along with thousands of others) for Christin Meeks who has cancer. I want this young beautiful girl to *live!* I believe nothing is impossible with God. Nothing.

Yes, I believe God hears prayer; God hears and answers. But the answer may be "yes," "no," or "wait." Not exactly what we expected.

There are some spiritual rumors that test my soul. Books, tapes, preachers saying that if I had enough faith, if I prayed the right prayer, if I "held on to my healing", if the people who prayed were *really* holy people, if, if, if . . . I would be physically healed. Toxic faith! One woman prayed for me, stood up and said, "Now you are healed. If you have REAL faith, stop taking your medication." What a torment. But I've realized these people (even if they're confused) come with love for me.

Jeff Cotter, the minister of our church, asked if he and some elders could come and pray. Of course I said yes. But as the Sunday afternoon approached, my chest tightened. Not strong enough to dress, I put on a pink robe and sat like a broomstick on a chair in the middle of my bedroom. As everyone filed in, they smiled and made easy conversation. But my words of thankfulness rolled awkwardly around in my mouth. "Well, let's pray," Jeff said. I squeezed my burning eyes shut.

The hands of these men and women rested on my back, shoulders, and head like a living blanket. Full of quiet passion, Jeff prayed. Their hands. Their wonderful hands. So much energy. Someone's hands felt hot on my back. My heartbeat slowed. My breath moved in and out like a gift. As people offered simple prayers, Love soaked my skin, soaking my soul. Jeff said, Amen, anointing my head with oil.

After they left, peace remained. I opened my worn red *Book of Common Prayer.*

> This is another day, O Lord. I know not what it will bring forth, but make me ready, Lord, for whatever it may be. If I am to stand up, help me to stand bravely. If I am to sit still, help me sit quietly. If I am to lie low, help me to do it patiently. And if I am to do nothing, let me do it gallantly. Make these words more than words and give me the Spirit of Jesus. [10]

I sucked the words into my flesh. I knew God could take lupus away, and perhaps one day He would. It didn't happen that Sunday. But through holy hands I experienced palpable love. I knew God loved me because I am. And that's the deepest healing I could ever desire.

Pray for yourself, ask others to pray. Pray for me, and Frances, I will pray for you.

Love,
Barbra Kay

TRUSTING THE MYSTERY

Journal
November 10, 1988

Yesterday I went to Christin's funeral. Her incredible parents chose to have an incredible celebration. The church was filled with people young and old. Everyone has been stretched by the life, death, and faith of this child.

These last months our whole community kept prayers for Christin on their breath. As she grew weaker, she saw only family and her best friend Amy. I kept in touch with Barbara, ready to do anything. Anything. But there was nothing more to do. We never finished <u>Lamper's Meadow</u>. We never finished our questions.

Through tears people asked each other why God took her. Christin of all people. So young. So exceptional. So much of her life unfinished. But reflecting on Christin, I think she did more living in her almost fifteen years than most people do in seventy.

During this illness she took over her life. She learned about her disease and helped make decisions about her treatment. She struggled with questions about life and death and God. She came to conclusions. She chose life every day, enjoying the things teens enjoyed—being with her friends, wearing Guess jeans, talking on the phone surrounded by stuffed animals and posters. She wrote letters to former teachers and friends about her faith. She campaigned for a camp for kids with cancer.

Pressed into maturity, she experienced a deep bond with her mother and father. She enjoyed little brother Tim. She formed a strong link with her brother Isaac. Rather than letting pain overtake her, she learned to meet pain. As her body became a wisp of a shadow, she radiated the soul of a giant.

Yes, no doubt, God saw Christin finished. Ready to go on with Him. Goodbye, Christin. We will cry for ourselves. We will cry for your mother and father and brothers. But you, my woman-child, you are safe with God.

Just as you believed, Jesus has healed you forever. And you have shown me how to trust the Mystery.

MINA

PRECIOUS EXISTENCE

Journal
December 5, 1988

What a difference one experience can make in your life. I decided to visit Ruth, a fiery octogenarian, who lives at the Lutheran Home (against her will) since she had a stroke. It would be good for me to think of somebody else for a change, and I thought she'd like the company. I knocked softly. She knew I was coming, so I opened the door. Ruth was sitting on her bed in a gray cotton jacket. The room was hot, but she had her feet covered with a blue wool blanket. Under her cap of thin short hair, she looked so small. I said I was coming in and she growled, "Well, I'm here. There's no other place I can be."

I tried to jolly her up, telling her I brought her a book and I thought she might like a poinsettia. She'd have none of it. "Can't see to read," she said. "And no plants! I can't take care of any plants. I just wish I could have a cat. But no animals in this place. It's like a prison."

I looked around her room. It was pleasant with a bath, kitchen nook, her antique four-poster bed and matching chest, a comfortable green rocker and fold-out couch with lots of pillows, small coffee table with Bible, cut glass candy dish, three black carved elephants. Tiny china bowls, cut glass tray, funny stuffed rabbit, hand-painted cups and saucers sat arranged on her corner glass shelves. I asked her about the family pictures hanging in dark walnut frames, and she lit up. "Born in Colorado," she told me. Her story unfolded. Strong youngster riding bareback in the mountains. Married and widowed early, she raised her son David and made her way through life, riding her horses and loving her people. Always farming, she had chickens and goats, raised tomatoes, beans, corn in the summer, pickled and canned and stored and froze for the winter. Coping. Being independent. Saying her mind. And these were her folks. Mother and father. Husband and son. And see her there, on the back of that wagon with all the hay. Used to help her husband bale when there weren't enough hands. And there.

There she is in front of her house in California. All painted white with red trim. And now? Good for nothing. Sitting in here. What for?

Ruth sighed. I hugged her, and told her I felt the same way lots of times. Her brown eyes stared at me through coke bottle glasses. I touched her hand and explained that when my illness gets mean, sometimes I'm in bed for months. But I've decided God is invested in our being—not just our doing.

She shook her white head. "Useless."

I told her I was leaving the poinsettia. I'd come back and water it.

On the way home I wondered about learning we are precious simply because we exist. My learning opportunity just came a little early. I want to see a lot of Ruth. We have things to teach each other.

MINA

TODAY IS THE FIRST DAY
OF THE REST OF YOUR LIFE

January 4, 1989

Dear Gary,

HAPPY BIRTHDAY! Do you realize you've now lived more of your life with me than you lived single. Scary!

Thank you for the effort you've put into our marriage. Thank you for trying this living arrangement. There have been some gifts in the separation. When I listen for your car pulling into the driveway on Friday nights, I feel excited. When I told you last week I was scared of my next treatment, I realized our nightly phone conversations free us to say things we might not say face to face. When I wrote to you about missing my job, I realized writing letters frees me to express feelings I can't say aloud. Yes, what I was so afraid of—our separation—has given us gifts.

For your birthday present I've decided to give you a funny present once a week. It may be a joke. It may be a funny story. It may be a hilarious movie. It may be me in a red wig. WATCH OUT!

Today is the first day of the rest of your life! May every day be filled with good. I'm glad you were born, Gary Minar. And I'm glad you're my husband. I love you.

Barbra

LOVE TALK

February, 16, 1989

Dear Frances,

Honey, your stress busters were great—especially "fly to Paris."
Let's get real! But after I read your letter I understood.

I'm not surprised that you and Paul are struggling because of
your last setback. I'd be surprised if you weren't. There are a lot of
emotional stages to get to acceptance. Denial, anger, grief. And
Gary and Paul have to go through them too. It takes a superhu-
man effort to keep any marriage growing, and add a life-threaten-
ing illness or disability and POW! You've got big problems. The
facts are scary. Seventy-five percent of marriages with these challenges end in divorce. It seems like chronic problems really spot-
light our weaknesses. Knowing that, we can walk into the rough
parts and try to strengthen our partnership.

I know you feel bad because Paul has to shop and cook and
take on extra kid duties after he's worked all day. I worry when I'm
down and extra responsibility falls on Gary. It seems the problems
are worse when we can't talk about things. Like fear. Fear that we
might lose each other. Fear that our marriage has changed. Our sex
life has changed. Our social life has changed. Our work life has
changed. Our financial picture has changed. Yes, it seems to me
we've got to talk and talk and talk. And that's so hard, because we
both want to avoid the pain. But talking is the surgery that will
open us up so we won't fester and explode. And by the grace of
God, talking together we might create a tested love that endures
all things.

I was talking about this with my friend Julie, who had a double
mastectomy last March and lost her hair from the chemo. She
needed affection desperately but felt so unattractive she shied away
from her husband. Finally she just blurted it out. "Dick, do I look
too ugly to touch?" He told her the truth. Getting used to her
body was hard. But he loved her deeply. She wasn't just a body

MINA

and he took her in his arms for the first time in months. She's a gutsy woman, that Julie. And she encourages me to be honest.

One thing about all this talking—it doesn't have to be about THE ILLNESS all the time. Good grief! I don't want my marriage to be disease focused Hey, honey! Maybe flying to Paris *is* a good idea. And if not Paris—have a picnic on your bed. Wear high heels with your pajamas. Paint your toenails yellow. Put perfume on your neck. Put soft music on your CD and push "repeat." Call Paul in beside you and lock the door. And, oh honey, talk with your hands.

I'll keep you in my prayers.

Fondly,
Barbra Kay

THE DAY OF GRACE

Journal
March 17, 1989

I had a rough night.

But today I feel the sweet spring wind at my back. I'm going to get out of bed, dress in lavender and dance the samba and eat jelly beans and drink white wine and call all my friends and wear my purple hat and go barefoot and throw rose petals in the street and kiss my cat and smile even when I sleep. I sold my book. <u>Unrealistic Expectations</u>. I did! Carole Streeter called from Victor Books, and Gary's so excited he bought me a Nancy Phelps watercolor of a woman standing in flowers. It's called "Grace."

Bless my young mom's group. It's hearing their stories, hammering out their questions, that pressed the words out of me. Oh, God, thank you for your tether. The restrictions I fought—being alone, being in bed, are the very things I needed to forge this writing. What was meant for evil, you used for good. You helped me find healthy work!

INTRUSION AT THE CROSSROAD

May 25, 1989

Dearest Katherine,

What an incredible graduation! Dad's popping his buttons bragging about you. Getting through college in four years is fantastic! Enclosed are some of the pictures we took. I never think we look alike except for our blue eyes, but baby, we have identical celebration grins!

Now here you are, poised to dive into life and knocked down with Epstein-Barr virus. But I'm enormously relieved your tests for lupus came back negative! Before you were born, no one thought there was any genetic link to lupus. Now there's information that puts daughters at a ten percent risk. But that means you have a ninety percent chance of being lupus-free.

You've been such a trooper! Finding doctors. Researching. Eating right. Resting and resting. I know you've been afraid and I've been afraid, too—and fighting guilt because I might have passed a gene combination on to you. Because of my history, I'm sure doctors will check again for lupus if you have any symptoms. But if something ever turns up, we can meet it together, just like we're going to meet this virus. Being healthy means working to be *whole* in body, mind, and spirit. And sometimes it's our limitations that wake us up! We begin to honor our bodies. We begin to relish life. We begin to depend on God.

Now here's my prescription. Throw confetti every day! Stomp through Sacramento in your dinosaur slippers. Kiss babies. Don't miss a sunset. Love somebody.

I'm here loving you,
MOM

Barbra Goodyear Minar

GOODBYE GUILT

Journal
May 10, 1989

Coming to Gary's house in Long Beach is a challenge. I have quiet during the day and can devise my own writing and resting schedule. But just as I sit down at the chrome kitchen table with my books and computer, the house begins whining, and I look up. A hodgepodge of worn garage couches and attic chairs sit in disarrayed lumps like faded old ladies who sag around their middles. The refrigerator groans. Vile smells hit when I open the door and look in bags of moldy hamburger and furry rotting oranges. The kitchen floor creaks as my feet stick to bits of coffee, sugar crumbs, and oil splashes. Sheets holler, "Change me!" The blinds cough dust when I pull them up. Mail and newspapers and dirt and clothes have accumulated from Gary and his roommates Doug and Chuck who share this place. Totally out of place, Doug's grand piano sits like a regal black queen in the corner of the living room. Everything's screaming, "Dust me, scrub me, vacuum me. You should, you ought to, you better, you lazy, ungrateful girl!"

Alert! Sounds like Cinderella's wicked stepmother yelling in my head. What's the deal? If I clean up all this mess, I'll be worn out with no energy for writing. With <u>Lamper's Meadow</u> finished, I have this idea for a new project. Yes, that's what I want to do. So goodbye guilt. I'll throw the spoiled stuff out of the refrigerator and then—I'm hittin' my computer and resting after lunch.

THE BLESSED ORDINARY

Journal
July 17, 1989

Tonight I unloaded a basket of clothes from the dryer and carried it to the bedroom. I buried my face in Gary's faded blue pajamas, smelling the warm clean cotton. I folded the worn work pants and shirt and laid them on the bed. I rolled matching socks together, pressed undershirts and shorts with my hand and stacked them on the bed. I remember folding clothes with my grandmother and mother. As a little girl, matching socks was my job. Carefully rolling from the toe and tucking the ball together with out stretching.My nose in dryer fluffed or line-dried clothes always soothes my body. The folding rituals soothes my soul.

Nothing spectacular happened today. The phone didn't ring. No children called with problems. Put on sunscreen and took an early walk with my dog. Talked to Gary about the dry weather. Watered the blue lobelia and white sweet alyssum on my porch. Watched the blue jays chasing the wrens away from the bird feeder. Fed and brushed my cat. Called Ann. Drank coffee with Francie. Opened my mail. Curled up in bed reading Frederick Buechner's Brendan. *Ate a peanut butter and banana sandwich for lunch. Did a load of wash. Wrote a four-line poem. A quiet day. A commonplace day.*

I wonder if too often I feel I haven't really lived unless there's been a crisis, high activity, pressure. God, help me seek the health of the hushed days of peace. The blessed days of the holy ordinary.

Barbra Goodyear Minar

LIVING IN COMMUNITY

Journal
December 3, 1989

Jenny and Mark invited me to baby Sarah's christening at the Episcopal church in Arroyo Grande. Morning light pouring through a stained glass window of the Shepherd and his lambs filled the church with red, blues and whites creating celebration. I slipped into the second row right behind the family. The somber two-month-old blinked tiny raisin eyes at me over her mother's shoulder. I studied her little face with skin as smooth as a pear. Black sprouts of hair poked up in shock. Perfect fingers tangled in her mother's long hair.

She was content, taking it all in until it was time for the christening and Jenny slipped Great Grandmother's baby bonnet on her head and tied the pink satin ribbon under her chin. Sarah howled. Godparents and grandparents stood with Jenny and Mark in front of the priest in his heavy black robe and bright red vestment, the new parents passing Sarah back and forth in her long white antique dress while she screamed, her little round face as red as a tomato. Jenny's eyes filled. I held my breath. Oh, don't cry, dear heart. Your baby's all right. You've waited so long for this moment.

"We present Sarah Elizabeth Michaels to receive the Sacrament of Baptism," said the godparent. The priest began. "Will you be responsible for seeing that the child you present is brought up in the Christian faith and life?" "We will, with God's help," said the parents and godparents.

The baby cried on. Then with huge hands he scooped the child from her father's arms and untied the bonnet.

Sarah grew suddenly still, as if she knew this was a holy time. "Sarah Elizabeth Michaels." The priest took water from the font. Baptizing her in the name of the Father, and of the Son, and of the Holy Spirit. Amen Then he lifted her to his chest, cradling her against his body. He prayed, and ignoring the whole congregation, he looked into her face and made the sign of the cross on her forehead. She stared up at him. Then gently straightening out the hem of her gown, he walked her up and down the long aisle. Sarah pursed up her lips. The congregation laughed and erupted in spontaneous applause.

This church had supported Jenny when she found out she was ill. They celebrated Jenny and Mark's wedding, and now the congregation had committed to support their adopted child. So much of life must be understood together. There's health in community.

Thank you, Sarah, for being. For your being is bringing great joy!

GOOD MEDICINE IS LOVING A DO

Journal
March 22, 1990

Today I took Happy to visit Ruth. As Happy sniffed the tulips and daffodils, I tugged her along the sidewalk to #17. Residents smiled and nodded along the way and let Happy's pink tongue wash their hands. Then we were stopped by an old man wearing a worn a tweed jacket and brown cowboy hat. Frail and bent, eyes to the ground he moved slowly in his walker. "Happy!" I jerked her back, afraid she might tip him over. "Well, hello fella." He reached for the dog and the walker rocked. He held on laughing and scrubbed Happy's ears with a gnarled hand. "Dang, I used to have me a pack a dogs," he said. "Never a lonely day, right fella?"

Happy's black tail thumped against the man's thin legs. "I love labs, myself. Best friends." He looked at me; his face brightened. I told him she's a youngster chewing up my slippers. He patted her wagging back end. "Dang, I miss havin' me a dog. You be a good Happy girl now! Yeah. I used to train dogs. Always had one ridin' in my truck." Looking at his bright old face, I promised we'd visit again.

Opening the door at Ruth's. The drapes were pulled shut. The stale room was hot. Ruth was slumped on her couch, legs covered with a brown and yellow afghan. "You're late." Her voice was gruff. "Somebody's here to see you," I said, pulling Happy in and trying to keep her tail from sweeping the knicknacks off the coffee table. Ruth scooted to the edge of her cushion and put both hands on the dog's back. "Good girl. Best girl." Her voice drifted into a whisper as she scratched Happy's head. Happy rolled over on her back, feet straight in the air and wiggled all over. Ruth laughed. "Oh, I keep treats in this place for the likes of you." She struggled to get up and made her way around the dog to her walker and scooted across the room while I held my breath afraid she'd fall in a heap. As Happy jumped up and followed Ruth to her cookie jar, the dog practically filled her entire apartment. "Yes, I do. Keep these cookies." She reached inside and pulled out a dog bone. "Keep hoping for real friends to come by. Here have another." Laughing and talking and clucking, Ruth fed Happy five cookies. After thirty minutes I was completely exhausted trying to keep Happy from knocking Ruth down. But Ruth was beaming. "Come back when you can," she said. "Sure like your dog there. You know I really miss having my cat."

As Happy and I drove home, I wished with all my heart that Ruth could have her cat. At eight-nine you ought to be able to have a cat if you want. One thing I do know. This dog carries pure happiness and I want to spread it around.

Barbra Goodyear Minar

WELCOME, OLD FRIEND

Journal
April 2, 1990

Gary's moving home. Three years and four months of commuting are behind us. What felt like an earthquake, shaking our home in two, turned out to be more foundation cement. Separated, I've grown stronger. Now I must readjust and save energy for Gary. I've gotten used to the solitary days. Now every morning the <u>Los Angeles Times</u> will be spread over the kitchen table. He'll bring home stories from the office. He'll "baby talk" the cat and throw the ball for the dog. He'll work on cars for his friends. He'll leave cigar butts in the garden. He'll buy the food. I'll cook the dinner. And before we eat we'll give thanks. Then sports and news will blare from the TV. Every night he'll hang his pants on the doorknob. I'll stop sleeping in my gray sweats and take my books and journal off his side of the bed, and he will sleep with me. Every night I'll see his care as he looks in my face. I'll be more truthful. Truthful about my emotions. And how my body feels. Not because Gary will always understand, but because it's healthier for me to share. I want to share and not expect. And hopefully we'll keep growing closer. Welcome home, my husband, my old friend. We're turning the page and our story goes on. Welcome home.

SHARING

Gary's head rested on his chest in his old brown leather chair tonight, sleeping through a TV western. There was no suitcase to pack with clean pants and shirts for the week. No three hour trip to Long Beach. Instead tomorrow he'll drive thirty-five minutes to his new job at Vandenberg.

He looked tired from all the details of moving back home. His forehead's mapped with lines and his dimples have deepened to creases down his cheeks. Yes, he looked tired. I gently shook his arm and told him it was time for bed. He jerked awake, opened his heavy eyes and smiled. "Have to eat some ice cream first. Have any chocolate chip?" Back in his chair he clinked the spoon loudly against the glass cup, scraping out the last precious sweet comfort, then got up and went to bed.

Long after he fell asleep, I lay beside him, my head under my pillow as he snored. With the familiar warm silk of his body against mine, my breathing steadied.

I was glad he transferred back here. And anxious, too. The bed I claimed during the week, the island I slept on with papers and books, now would be straightened for him. My early bedtimes would change. I had to make dinner, clean dishes, sit in the den before bed. One thing I'd learned during our separation. Sleep was as vital to my health as food.

When Gary's snoring swelled, I poked him with my foot. He kept snoring. I reshifted the pillow around my ears. I was glad he was home, but I'd gotten used to the five days of independence I'd never had before. And, of course, he had too.

I rolled over and put my hands on his back, feeling the inhale and exhale of his exhausted sleep. "You're snoring," I whispered. There was silence and then sound. Bless you, husband. I rolled out of bed and walked down the dark hall to Katherine's old bedroom, crawled in bed and shivered between the cold sheets.

FIFTY-YEAR-OLD CHILD

June 7, 1990

Dear Dad,
Thanks so for my birthday phone tonight. Can you believe you have a fifty-year-old child? I loved having you tell me about you and Mom going fishing the morning of my birth and how you got the model T stuck. I can just see Mom in labor with her huge belly rubbing against the wheel as she steered while you, slopping around in the mud, frantically pushed the car! I'm sure glad you managed to free us so I wasn't born at the fishing hole.

I know you've worried so about me these past years. But I want you to know that even on the worst days I've been grateful I am experiencing life. It's all a gift.

I've been reflecting on my story—the high moments: sleeping the first night in my own room at ten, winning the seventh grade poetry contest, pulling from my Christmas box the black and blue plaid taffeta formal Mother made for me, holding my first naked newborn on my jelly stomach. And the low moments: breaking up with my first love at seventeen, hearing I had lupus at twenty, crushing under the weight of mother's death when I was twenty-two, living with the agony of Jeff's drug addiction. It's the mix of experiences that's thickened my soul.

Oh, Dad, thank you for grappling with your young life on the Kansas wheat farm, for pressing through the depression to finish Friend's University, for marrying your college sweetheart without a penny between you, for driving from Kansas to California to see the Redwoods in 1939, for having the courage to have children, for fighting in World War II and for suffering through the torment after you came home, for building a home and providing food and clothes and medical care by going to work faithfully through the years, for remarrying after mom died and starting a new life.

Without the tough times I wouldn't have seen your courage. Without seeing your pain, I would have collapsed when pain first seared me. Without observing your grief, I wouldn't have known how to cry and still walk. And all the high times big and small. The eloquent toasts you give at family weddings, the look when I put your first grandson in your arms, the prayers you prayed daily over baked chicken and mashed potatoes, the boyish laughter when you skunk me at Hearts. Oh, yes, all of it's good. So good. It's fodder for life, and my first night of being fifty years old I want to honor it all. I want to sing to it all! My history is my fertilizer for my future. Now I hope something new will spring up from my land.

Dad, never stop sharing your wisdom. It's truly my inheritance.

I love you!
Barbra Kay

P.S.

Happy birthday to me.
Happy birth—day—to—me!
Happy birthday to me!!!
I grew up to be 50!

LIFE WITH A VIEW

Journal
November 10, 1990

After pulling out my black suitcase from under the bed and opening it on the floor, I lay down. If I didn't have the energy to pack, how would I ever hold up driving ten hours to Yosemite? This afternoon, changing from my tennis shoes to slippers because of swollen ankles, I wondered how I was going to walk? Maybe I should just call the whole trip off. But then Gary would be so disappointed. I dug into my personal pharmacy and filled a zippered case with medication and vitamin and herbs I might need. The mountains would be beautiful with yellows and reds. I packed my camera. Probably cold, too. I packed sweats, sweaters, jeans and a long wool skirt and then crawled into bed

The house was cold, so I buried in blankets. The coldest place I ever lived was years ago in Wyoming. I remembered leaving the Cheyenne hospital after Steven was born with strict instructions from the pediatrician to take Steven outside every day. It really got cold in Wyoming! The Indians said the Cheyenne Winter Wind dumped snow from her skirt and shook ice from her hair. But every day, no matter what the weather, I put on boots and coats and wool scarf and zipped Steven in his blue snow suit to go outside. Sometimes, wrapped like mummies in blankets, we stood in the snow blowing tiny clouds from our mouths on the doorstep. There were always marvels to see—ducks flying, animal tracks, long icicles, and in the sky beyond the confines of my small house I saw the skirts of Winter Wind. No matter what had perplexed my day, in that brief adventure outside, shivering in my coat, shifting my wiggling child, I felt like singing to the Creator.

Yes, going to Yosemite will be good. Even if I have to stand on the doorstep and look.

I pulled myself out of bed and found my old brown boots.

HUGGING TREES

November 12, 1990

Dear Frances,

Guess what! We're in Yosemite. I'm taking a rest while Gary goes hiking. I've been able to walk some through yellow leaves of the black oaks and catch sight of squirrels, fox, and deer. You can feel the quiet excitement of fall and the promise of snow, as if the sky were pregnant and will deliver white only in her known moment. We walked the path from Laurel Lodge to the falls and back, poking along with our walking sticks and collecting leaves. And honey, we ate big hot fudge sundaes with nuts and cherries for lunch.

Later we drove to the great Redwood trees in Mariposa Grove, and I was overcome. Imagine a tree twenty-seven hundred years old! I walked *inside* of trees, looking up into dark sky caves. I put my hands on rough thick bark, blacked from fires. One hundred forty types of insects live in the trees, but nothing but an axe brings the mighty forest kings down What majesty!

To think I almost backed out of this trip! Even though I have pain, it doesn't compare to the joy of being part of life with those trees. What if I'd never held such mystery in my arms or let it hold me? It reminds me once again that ,while my illness is part of my life, it doesn't define me. No, some holy Power beyond myself defines me. The same Power that defines the redwoods. I think I understand what Einstein meant when he wrote "The most beautiful thing we can experience is the mysterious." We leave in the morning for home, but I'm not the same person who came.

Love,
Barbra Kay

MIXED INHERITANCE

Journal
December 8, 1990

What else can happen to Jeff? My poor son. Whenever I hear his voice on the phone I feel a cold wind blowing in my ear. He called this morning with another blow. Now he's been diagnosed with discoid lupus from the red, scaly lesions on his scalp and arms. Right away I looked it up in my lupus book and read that few people with discoid go on to have systemic lupus. But why does he have to deal with this when he has so much else on his plate?

Guilt draped over my heart. Washing the breakfast dishes, my mind wandered through the bubbles, deep into the water where I saw Jeff's sad eyes staring up at me. No! I won't think about it. Pulling up the sheets on the bed, I remembered tucking covers around his child body and suddenly saw his arms covered with red lesions. Brushing my teeth, I lost myself in the mirror and saw scarring and bald spots on the top of his head. I filled the basin with cold water and splashed my face until I could wake up. I must remember I am not responsible for placing the genetic makeup in Jeff's body. I am not in charge of the mysterious communion of sperm and egg connecting and exploding, multiplying through the seconds, making his form. The gifts and the flaws. They are a part of his journey.

I called Jeff back. "Did your doctor tell you what medications to use?" He caught the breathiness in my voice. "Don't worry." He sounded firm "Don't worry, Mom, I watched you deal with it. I can too."

Once more, God. Help me let go. He can walk through this. Courage, too, came through the generations to his genetic code.

VICTORY WOMEN

January 10, 1991

Dear Frances,

It's 1991 and we're still kicking! Not only that, but this year we're going to grow even more.

Now, I've got some ideas for the New Year. We've both got a puzzle to solve. We're supposed to exercise, but sometimes we feel worse afterwards, so we quit. Right? Right! Well, I've been sloshing this around in my mind, doing a lot of reading, and I've decided that I am going to exercise every single day that I can. Sometimes when I think of exercise, I already feel defeated. My daydreams spin with Julie Jazzercise in her shiny leotard who dances laps around the gym and does one thousand sit ups to rock music while I'm still getting my tennis shoes tied. I HATE HER. Still, I know I've got to exercise.

Oh, I hear you moaning. Hang on. First I'm exchanging the word EXERCISE for the word MOVEMENT. Does that help?

I look at it this way. Maybe some days all I can do is move my fingertips and wiggle my nose, but I know movement is the most basic expression of being *alive.* And, honey, you know how I love being alive. Oh yes!

Saying I've got to *exercise* every day sounds like a horror, but saying I'm going to *move* every day sounds like life. Maybe this is just a trick of my mind, but that's okay. And I've decided not to be in a hurry. Year after year I get started, overdo, collapse and give up. This time I'm going to pace myself.

The first thing I'm going to tackle (don't laugh) is my breathing. I do know some breathing techniques from pain management, and I could practice them every day. Just moving those old lungs in and out. And I found these gentle stretches I can do in bed before I get up. I'm sending you a copy. And what do you think about this idea? If it's not *fun*, I'm going to try something else. The idea is just to keep MOVING.

One thing that's important is to keep away the competition. I have to confess, watching Julie Jazzercise made me feel like a dolt because I was comparing. Well, that won't work. I'm going to reward myself for every effort. Even if it's stretching two minutes every day for a week. And when I feel good enough, I'm going to put on jazz and dance like a wild thing around my bedroom.

Send me your ideas. This could be 1991, the Year of Victory Women!

Love,
Barbra Kay

A MELANCHOLY SONG

Journal
March 11, 1991

I'm losing my hair. And for some reason it's jogging early memories. Mother brushing and braiding my long blond hair as I sat on the kitchen stool. I remember, too, the first time I washed and rinsed that long hair in the bathtub by myself at six. How splendid I felt being in charge of the shampoo as I squeezed a blob into my hand and scrubbed my head and rinsed my hair under the metal spigot until a strand would squeak. Then came nights of the pin curls twisted in paper held with bobby pins pressing against my scalp, and those metal curlers, and pink soft curlers I slept in. The hair cut short, the hair grown out. The barrettes, rubber bands, and ribbons. Pony tails, French twists, page boys. Hair spray, conditioners, gels. The permanent that fried my hair into frizz the day of the senior prom. Streaking my darkening hair with blond, tinting it red, bleaching it white. Looking in the car mirror to check my hair, running to the ladies room to check my hair, slipping out my compact to check my hair.

Now my thick brown and gray mane is coming out in big clumps. When I wash it, hair clogs the shower drain. When I brush it, my brush needs to be cleaned. When I sleep, it falls out on my pillow. I find myself trying not to touch my head, thinking my hair might stay in longer. I knew the medication could cause hair loss, but when it didn't happen right away, I thought I was exempt. And anyway, I told myself, losing my hair would be a small price to pay for getting well. A small price. But now that it's happening, I feel nude. Exposed as if someone keeps walking into my bathroom, catching me without a towel.

Thumbing through the yellow pages looking for a store that sold wigs to people like me, I suddenly felt like a note in a melancholy song. A song of all the brave people who have lost their covering. I will sing along with you. And I will recover.

Barbra Goodyear Minar

PUSHING THE LIMITS

Journal
May 8, 1991

I'm discouraged about my writing. <u>Lamper's Meadow</u> has been rejected by sixteen publishers. My visit to Steve and Kathy's in El Granada was the refreshing break I so needed. Every morning while I drank my tea I sat at their kitchen window looking through the eucalyptus trees at the ocean. Having Katherine with us was an extra plus. But the best part was the surprise.

Hearing excitement and energy in her voice, I knew Kathy had something special planned. The morning of the surprise she asked me if I thought I could ride her horse, California. She had borrowed horses for Katherine and herself. Ignoring my noodle legs, I said sure. She encouraged me, saying we'd go early and that the ride was shady and easy.

After a skimming sleep filled with runaway horses, I got up and painted myself with thick sunblock, dressed in long sleeves, pants and wide-brimmed hat. This cowgirl was ready. And if anything happened—well, Katherine would be sympathetic and Kathy was a nurse, so . . . We drove the jeep to the stables and, while the girls fed and groomed and saddled the horses, I looked for droppings from the barn owl, collected eucalyptus pods, sat on a hay bale watching mice adventures, and poked around the ancient barn. I ignored my complaining joints and my nervous imaginings.

I rubbed California, fed her a carrot and told her to WALK. Then with coaching from Kathy, I put my foot in the stirrup and grabbed the saddle horn. It was hard to swing up and stretch my legs across California's black and white back. My legs were shaking from the effort. "Good going, Mom," Katherine yelled, "Good going!" patting the horse's flank. California danced to the left. I grabbed the reins in my sweating hands and followed the narrow trail behind Katherine and Kathy. I wondered if the surprise was that I'd never make it back home.

As we came out of the trees we could see cloud mountains painted across the May sky. We rode up a hill and stopped. Glistening on our left, the giant Pacific chopped into wet light from the wind and sun. The shocking beauty froze the moment. Even the horses stood still.

"It's not too far now," Kathy said, finally turning her horse down into a canyon. I pressed my trembling legs into California's belly so I wouldn't fall off as we trotted behind. Where were we going?

Suddenly we came out into a field of blinding gold. Wild daffodils! My breath caught in my chest. In that splendor all the storms in my life seemed to vanish. The girls got down from their horses into the flowers. As they took long-legged strides, the sun washed their hair with light. I lifted my leg over the saddle with my hands, slid off California and sat in the field. As the horse nosed around and grazed, I lost myself looking into the ruffled face of a daffodil. The elegant flower looked like a sun bonnet on a tall young lass. This perfection sprang from a small dark bulb that had waited for its growing through winter, through rain, through warming earth. Going through a process to explode into its full self. And who does this wild field bloom for? Rarely does anyone see the glory of this hidden place. I suppose the daffodils bloom just for God's pleasure.

Katherine and Kathy came back with arm loads of yellow. I picked two large bunches for myself. On the way home I knew I had pushed my limits. I was too tired. I had gotten too much sun. I had pushed my limits. And deep inside I felt healthier than ever. Thanks, Kathy. Thanks for the fantastic surprise.

Barbra Goodyear Minar

A SUNRISE OF THANKFULNESS

Journal
November 30, 1991

Last month my body hurt in the night. Depression had his head on my pillow. And when the phone rang early, I gave a grumpy hello. It was Steve and Kathy. They wanted to tell us—and in a rush the news came out. They are expecting a baby in late May. After trilling words of delight, I hung up the phone and lay back on my pillow—alone. That devil Depression was gone!

The life cycle rotates on. Birth and death and birth. Oh, babies are born every day. I read birth announcements in the paper, get them in the mail, hear the good news from my friends. It always warms me on the inside. But this is a different baby. A grandbaby. My grandbaby.

There've been times I prayed to live long enough to see my children grown. I've prayed for the future of my grandchildren. But I dared not dream of knowing my grandchildren. But look! Here's one coming.

At Thanksgiving we got to see the video of "baby's first pictures"— the ultrasound. Kathy pointed out the baby's heart, and once we got our bearings, Gary and I sat on the floor near the TV and ran the tape over and over watching the tiny arms and legs, the spreading fingers. Steven tapped his finger on the screen, and we laughed. No doubt about it. Grandbaby is a boy. What a marvel!

There's always something to be grateful for: my buttered wheat toast in the morning, a cool breeze in July, smoke coming out of our white brick chimney, snapshots of my friends stuck on the refrigerator, unexpected notes in the mail, a good day's writing, a hot cup of lemon tea with milk and sugar. Thankful living is a whole, centered way to live. But sometimes there comes a sunrise of thankfulness that crowds your whole body. Thankfulness that blows away the fog mist and wings you off the ground. Thankfulness that wets your eyes and fills your mouth with prayer. Thank you, God. For this grandbaby coming.

AM I CRAZY?

December 22, 1991

Dear dear Jenny,

Here it is Christmas, and as usual the rush pushes me around like a wild wind. I started decorating the tree last night after you phoned. As I hung the ornaments and the tinsel, I kept hearing your sweet voice asking, "Do you think I'm crazy?"

First let me say, *you are not crazy!* The strange things you're encountering are your experience of lupus. Sometimes it's hard to tell my doctor certain things that are bothering me—especially when he doesn't seem to understand. A few years ago I started feeling a crawling numbness on my face and scalp; it was difficult to describe. The sensation burned and tingled. I was scared. In the night words like meningitis, paralysis, and stroke blinked on and off like neon lights. I worried about my family. What would they do if I had big time central nervous system problems? When I asked Dr. Gerber what it was, I was close to tears. He checked me over. "I think you have peripheral neuropathy. You don't need to worry." He wrote a few things on his pad and told me to see him in six weeks. Six weeks! What might happen to me in six more weeks? He must not understand. My face was numb! My arms were numb! I couldn't ask him anymore questions. The diagnosis sounded so terrible! The next appointment I told him how stressful this was for me.

Doctors want to "fix" whatever is wrong. But, Jenny, with chronic diseases that's often impossible, so when we complain and the doctor can't help, sometimes he passes it off. Also, when we bring in information he's unfamiliar with, occasionally our doctor may feel threatened. He might give us the feeling we don't know what we're talking about. After all, he's the one with medical training. We leave feeling we haven't been heard. And not being validated, we feel a little crazy.

Dear heart, BELIEVE in yourself. And find a support group. That's what I did when I had such an unsettling experience. The first group meeting I felt tongue tied and awkward. I almost decided not to go back. But the next week I was able to share how the neuropathy scared me. One redheaded woman named Sally pulled her chair beside me and covered my cold hands with hers. "I got that same weird crawling on my face. The good news is neuropathy ain't gonna kill us. The bad news is it's like a ghost that won't leave. Always hangin' around." I laughed and I think it was at that moment my heart stopped shivering. I love this saying: "God gives us the ingredients for our daily bread, but He expects us to bake it. "Maybe like me, you might find some of those ingredients in an encouraging group.

I'll talk to you after the holidays. In the meantime we can celebrate together in spirit. The Baby Jesus of Christmas is not a babe in a fairy tale. He is God. And He is with you.

Blessings,
Barbra

NEW INSIGHT

Journal
January 20, 1992

I guess I've known for twenty years I had cataracts from taking pred-nisone, and it didn't concern me much until these last few months. Suddenly things changed. I kept closing my right eye to check the left eye. I honestly couldn't read the big road signs anymore. Couldn't read bill-boards, for heaven sake. When Dr. Winthrop checked my eyes and sched-uled surgery, I wasn't surprised. He would do the left eye first and the right later. He told me he'd be taking the old lens out and giving me a lens implant. He walked me to the front desk, promising I'd see better than ever.

Seems like half the world has had cataract surgery and everyone said it was a "piece of cake." But hey! It was my eye this time. What if I got an infection, what if something happened in surgery? I love my eyes!

Gary drove me to St. Frances Hospital and stayed by my side, ner-vously patting my hand and frowning. We were home within a few hours. Wearing a metal patch taped over my eye, I was awkward even walking down steps. I never realized the depth perception two eyes gave me. I missed my eye.

The next morning Dr. Winthrop removed the patch and put drops in my eye. I rested my chin on the "light machine" as he peered into my eye, telling me cataract surgeries used to have long recoveries. Patients had to lie perfectly flat without moving their head for months. He pulled back and smiled. My surgery was perfect. Just perfect! Then he had me read the chart. I could see!

So donning giant dark glasses, I rode with Gary up the San Marcos Pass towards Solvang. When we slowed down behind a car pulling a boat over the mountain, I was glad. I wanted to see, see, see. The fog had burned away and as we took the first curve, the view spread from the bottom of the mountains out to the ocean. Santa Barbara glittered with bits of vivid red, yellow, and intense plum and sweeps of green running into the power-blue Pacific. *Huge clouds connected across the sky like mysterious moving islands. I'd forgotten that radiant white.*

I closed my watering eye and opened it again. Yes, that was it. I'd been seeing everything through a yellow gauze curtain for years. So slowly had the brilliance slipped away that I got used to the dulling of color and form. Now the gauze had been removed from my window and I could really see.

I wonder how much of my life has gotten covered with a film. How many things have faded from my awareness because I've forgotten what it's really like to "see." The three-year-old boy catching his first frog at the Santa Ynez River, the alcoholic man slouching in front of the Maverick, the young lovers touching noses in the rose garden at the Santa Barbara Mission. God, help me see all of life so I can truly be alive.

WIND IN MY SAILS

April 11, 1992

Dear Carolyn,

You doll! When Fancy Flowers delivered the basket of pink tulips and balloons, I flipped. Thanks for celebrating this wonder with me! After all the work, the tears, the rejections, the depression and the stubborn decisions to keep trying, I can actually hold *Lamper's Meadow* in my hand. It looks as though I have a six months' window to promote my baby and that's about it. If it takes off, you're in luck. If not—well—the book gets dumped and the words die in their paper tomb. That's scary.

I learned some things the hard way with *Unrealistic Expectations*. There's no way I have the energy (or the money) to peddle my book door to door. I have to do what I can by phone and letter. But I know one thing. I have a whole adventure ahead. I'll learn more about bookstores and libraries and marketing. I'll meet new people and give away my gift. And if it excites one child all the effort will be worth it. Working at something I love and exploring new directions makes me feel the wind filling my sail.

Oh, Carolyn, I never thought I'd write a book! And I never would have focused my active life if lupus hadn't changed my direction. It's as if I planned to travel to Africa to see wild elephants and tigers and ended up in Alaska ice fishing one hole instead. I could spend my days crying because I never got to take a safari. But I think I'll keep exploring this cold exciting land of long light and raw beauty. I guess no one really gets to dictate the terms of life, but what matters is how we live with our challenges.

No one really writes alone. I thank you with all my heart for the many times you invited me to sink into you like a favorite armchair when I was so discouraged and you held me with love until I patted away my discouraged tears and got back to the words. I wrote so much of this "with you."

Fondly,
Barbra

P.S. Keep your fingers crossed. Victor Books is looking at *Close Connections*. I'm sending you a copy of *Lamper's Meadow*—with all my love.

NEWBORNS

June 3, 1992

Dearest Steven,

Being with you the past week, I was exactly where I was supposed to be. Waiting. Touching Kathy's stretched stomach. Cooking the dinner. Setting the table. Clearing the table. Drying the pots. Trimming the violets. Washing the sheets. Folding the socks. Praying the prayers for mercy and safety and health as I worked. The graceful rhythm moved like the minute hand ticking off the sacred moments of waiting. Waiting to be initiated into the last trimester of my life by becoming a grandmother.

Yesterday morning wiping orange juice off the counter, I flashed back to your birth thirty-one years ago. The imprint in my cells from the pain and fear and ecstasy rushed through me. The feeling of pressure and push, the sounds of my groans and breaths, the smells of body and baby, the sight of you male, red, and crying. Sensing this holy squirming creation resting on my chest. It was all there in my mind.

Then finally last night we dressed and drove to the hospital. My whole self darted back and forth between Kathy's low moans and your concern. Through those seven hours in the delivery room with you and Kathy and her mom, Pat, God put excitement in my arms and legs, as if He played jazz into my bones.

Finally, just before 7:00 a.m., with all of us bubbling encouragement to Kathy, I watched the crowning. My heart thundered when the doctor suddenly rolled her stool close to the action and said she was removing the umbilical cord from around the baby's neck. Then Kathy gave one last intense push, and with a rush of water and blood, Christopher Steven Minar was breathing in the world. The room was electric—all of us laughing, crying and cooing. I took pictures of you cutting the cord and then focused on

Kathy. Oblivious of the lights and the people, she tucked her infant under her chin and closed her eyes in divine rest. In moments Pat held the baby and then, before he was twenty minutes old, you put Christopher into my arms. I could barely see him through the water of all grandmothers coming out of my eyes. So many births in that room: you a newborn father, Kathy a newborn mother, Pat and I newborn grandmothers. Our lives changed forever because of newborn Christopher. I know every birth, however ordinary, is extraordinary. Here against my old breast I held the holy once again.

As you left the delivery room, taking Christopher to weigh and measure in the nursery, I watched you through the glass partition. With your wide palm under his tiny head you unwrapped him and examined his feet and legs, his arms and long fingers. As you bent over this child, your brown eyes huge, I could see you talking to him. And when he clutched your finger, I saw your heart spilling out over his body. I saw your life being given away. There I was, watching my own cycle of life. My firstborn with his firstborn.

May God bless Christopher Steven. May all of his days be filled with awareness and the joy of being created.

Love,
Mom

THE TUNE WITHOUT WORDS

Journal
July 3, 1992

I need something to grab my mind and whistle hope back into my ears. I admit the last two weeks have been hard. Having to increase my medicine. Having to deal with odd symptoms. Fear in his black top hat and spats sat on the end of my bed, flipping through my thick medical chart, shaking his head and sighing. I almost sat up to ask, "What do you think it means? What's going to happen tomorrow?" Suddenly I caught myself. Here I go stirring up past horrors and making up future doom. VICTORY WOMAN! LIVE IN THE MOMENT!

I called Margy. "HELP!" was about all I could get out. In an hour she came by, arms filled with a picnic basket, a vase of lavender angel face roses, a gift wrapped in metallic purple paper.

Her dark eyes snapped and she smiled like an eight-year-old telling me to open my package fast! Ripping off the paper, I found the funniest pair of slippers. Knit black and white Mary Janes with a gold buckle and white socks. "We're going to have a party. Put them on." She clapped her hands "Oh, the're so funny. I wish I'd gotten some for me!" Then she threw a huge blue and white checkered table cloth over the bed and began setting out Greek olives, crackers, brie cheese, fresh tomatoes with basil, french bread and butter. She unloaded two china plates and silverware, long stemmed crystal glasses and a bottle of sparkling water. What a feast! As I nibbled at my crackers, I ate from her joy and drank in her compassion. We laughed when Prissy made a dash at the "picnic table." I stood up and made one twirl in my new Mary Janes. "I have one last present." Margy handed me a book. I turned it over. Love, Medicine & Miracles by Bernie Siegel. "You're in it. Start reading chapter eight." Margy swept away all the crumbs and dirty dishes, gave me a hug and left as magically as she had come.

Propped on my pillows I turned to chapter eight :" Becoming Exceptional." It started with

Hope is the thing with feathers

Barbra Goodyear Minar

that perches in the soul,
And sings the tune without the words
And never stops at all.

Emily Dickinson

Margy had helped me take a breath to hum that tune. And what do you know! That breath had blown Fear away with his hat in his hand.

INA

SURPRISED BY DEATH

Journal
August 6, 1992

At 1:20 p.m. today Gary's mother was killed. Evelyn died in a car accident. Broadsided by a teenage girl running a red light. Everyone's in shock, losing this powerful family matriarch. Last night I had a strong desire to call her. After a long chatty talk, laughing at old family stories, sharing new family happenings, I put Gary on the phone. I'm thankful I followed my intuition. I got to tell her I loved her. I got to say goodbye.

We had a long history, this strong woman and I. When Gary and I announced our marriage plans, she hung up the phone. I thought I could win her over, but she and I had to live out the rough edges. My mother-in-law pushed my buttons, insisting I should wallpaper my dining room, buying me an old gas stove that nearly blew up my kitchen, gossiping about her sister-in-law Josephine. But over the years she told me the deep windy stories: riding the milk truck to get home from her grandma's because she was homesick, making drapes to support her mother during the depression, working at a bakery while she was pregnant with the twins, taking on three love-starved stepsons when she remarried. Through these stories she let me into her soul.

I wasn't ready for this death. Evelyn's mother lived to be ninety-seven. Evelyn was feisty and healthy at eighty-two. I thought we had plenty of relationship time. What a reminder. All of us have a surprise ending to our earth story.

So today is the day I will look into the faces of my people. Today is the day I can drink in their being. I think I'll go call my dad.

Barbra Goodyear Minar

PLAY ONCE A DAY

December 8, 1992

Dear Frances,

Oh, honey, are you in trouble sending out Christmas cards on December 1st! Did you intend to give me the gift of envy for Christmas or what? Well, never mind. I'm skipping the whole deal and sending out Valentine's cards in February. Ain't that a grand idea? It's part of my "stress-less" Christmas plan.

I loved hearing about the bird sanctuary you've developed out your bedroom window. I never thought about being an "inside" birder. Bird feeders, birdbath, bird books and record books—what a great hobby. Since the Gulf Coast is such a fly-through to the islands, no telling how many birds you'll identify. I hope you enjoy the binoculars I've sent. My brother's a birder and he knew just what you needed. Small and light!

You'll never believe what I did this fall. I led a women's retreat. One morning I was coughing from bronchitis and asthma when I answered the phone and heard this cheery voice saying, "I'm Marcia Means calling from Lake Avenue Congregational Church in Pasadena." It's a huge church and I wondered what sort of fund raiser this could be! I kept coughing, and this woman went right on. "Our retreat committee read your book *Close Connections* and would like you to be our fall speaker." Well, honey! I wheezed out a "my goodness!" And started laughing. It seemed impossible.

I was in bed the whole month before the retreat, but I wrote and practiced my talks. Then the day before I was to leave, Dr. Gerber called to say my T cell count was thirty three and I must stay out of crowds. I sure didn't tell him my plans. Ann and Rebecca drove me to Canyon Meadows at Lake Hughes, and by cracky, with everyone's prayers and physical support, I was able to give four talks and spend time encouraging individual women. I had a wonderful, wonderful time. Spending the next month recovering was a small price to pay for such a gift. It was worth *everything*.

MINA

Honey, I've got this terrific idea. In 1993 let's come up with all the ways we can PLAY. Your birding counts. I bought myself a Christmas gift—a necklace with a tiny purple bottle of bubble juice and wand in the lid. I'm instantly ready to puff bubbles from my bed! It's my inspiration for my one New Year's resolution. *Play at least once a day!*

> May Christmas always be in your heart,
> Barbra Kay

P.S. Being a Grandmother is delicious!!!

ELASTIC PLANNING

Journal
January 7, 1993

And so I go into another year. It seems good to make goals. But to be realistic about handling lupus I must plan with some elastic in my soul, ready to be flexible and creative to reach my destination.

All morning I tried to get back to writing. Today was my deadline to START working on an article for <u>Guidepost</u>. Promptly at 9:00 a.m. I got to my desk, but my arms felt stiff. My brain was like a block of ice. My fingers froze on the computer keyboard. Trying to force words to appear on the screen I wrote vanishing sentences. I kept checking the clock as the morning flew by. Nothing. Nothing. Barbra, write. This is the perfect day. Company's gone. Gary's at work. As I straightened the books, counted my pencils, checked my pens for ink, Guilt grew a beard and moaned at me from my monitor. After dragging to the kitchen and making myself a third cup of tea, I sat back down and made a declaration. "YOU WILL STOP MESSING AROUND AND WRITE!" Guilt shook his finger and nodded. I started again.

Just as I was about to beat myself for fiddling with an old stack of mail, a warm rain started falling in my brain. The ice melted down just enough to think fresh. I needed to stop whipping myself and lie down. My body was trying to tell me to scratch the day's plan. Do something different, like take a nap. Call a friend. Read a joke. Watch the birds. Blow bubbles.

I turned off the computer and kicked off my tennis shoes. Just as I stretched out on my bed, Guilt hung over my face, his long dirty beard brushing my nose. He opened his mouth to start a lecture, but I shut my eyes and put a soft pillow over my head. Sleep put a million miles between us. And the strangest thing—I woke with ideas and words rolling around in my mind.

LOSING MY LIFELINE

Journal
January 30, 1993

I heard it last week from a friend. I didn't believe it. But Dr. Gerber told me during my visit today. He accepted a medical opportunity in Los Angeles. He's leaving. I couldn't grab his words whipping around the office about how he's enjoyed working with me, his hopes for my health in the future. He's leaving. He's leaving. After seventeen years as my lifeline. He's leaving. I said I was happy for him. I held my chin up. Grandma Goodyear said holding your chin up kept you from crying. But tears leaked out. Dr. Gerber took a tissue and wiped them away. I lifted my chin higher. Prescriptions, yes. Referral to another specialist, yes. Copy of my records, yes. A handshake. A hug.

Breathe, Barbra, breathe.

Past the nurses who squeezed my hand. Past the office staff who said we'll miss you. Past patients in the waiting room who would hear the same news. He's leaving.

Once on the sidewalk, I clutched my coat against the biting wind, walked stiffly to my car and slid across the seat, buckled up, started the engine and drove out of the parking lot. The street was a blur. The cars, the stop lights, the people.

Breathe, Barbra, breathe.

Barbra Goodyear Minar

TRUSTING AND LETTING GO

Journal
July 14, 1993

How deep I must go today. Deep into God. Trusting Him to hold me because I cannot stand. Trusting He knows all past and future. And that He is in control. When I sense the fragile stream of breath between me and death, I sense my tiny bits of dust. And I turn to the One who created me. Gave me body. Gave me spirit.

How can I know my body and my spirit? I know my body through pain when I cut my finger chopping onions, through hunger when I smell the pot roast cooking, through touch when I stroke Gary's face. I know my spirit through ache when I want to be understood, through hunger when I long for love, through yearning when I search for meaning. I know my spirit restless and stretching. What will it be like when my spirit is released from this worn container? It's a mystery. But who better to entrust my body and spirit to than my Maker. Yes, even in my death I will trust God to continue my life. And while I still have this priceless earth-life, I will search for God with all my heart. And I will find Him, for He is everywhere.

Like a November leaf
clinging to the elm branch
whipped by fall winds
I fear being ripped
from the limbs
of my home
But the moment will come
in a snap
and I shall be carried
in the arms of your Breath
into the holy world
of forever

MAPPING MEDICAL STRATEGIES

August 30, 1993

Dear Frances,

I've really had to face a transition. Dr. Gerber left in June. Oh, honey, you'd understand my grief. It feels as if the major link in my health care chain broke and the chain fell apart. I met with the new doctor Dr. Gerber suggested. The first visit was alright. As he examined me, he told me about his family and looked over the recent entry in my thick chart. But right away he wanted to take me off some medicine I've relied on. I was scared. I told myself, Okay. Just take it slow. I can do this. I have to do this. But last week at the follow-up appointment, he didn't remember my case. If my lupus flares, *where* is *my* doctor?

Yesterday when I asked my young dermatologist one more question on my list, she looked at her watch and said we had to hurry. She was allowed only fifteen minutes a patient! How can doctors be expected to practice medicine with such limitations? How can patients be expected to deal with their issues in a rush. Frances, we are *really* going to have to educate ourselves! And be our own best medical advocates.

Recently, Margy invited a few women together to discuss health challenges. Most were well women wanting to stay healthy. As we drank our tea, we passed around articles and and books. We exchanged doctor recommendations and info on breast cancer research, inner healing ideas, exercises and healthy diets, and plenty of encouragement all round. And after all the talk, Margy offered to be there if one of us needed help during an illness. This set us into more discussion with promises of incredible support.

Oh, Frances, when we were growing up, all these things used to be done by families; but today with fractured homes or long distant relatives we need to nurture a family of good friends. After all, who will walk the hospital corridors during surgery? Who will ask the doctor for the prognosis? Who will watch the dog, buy groceries, help run down insurance claims? Who will helps us laugh? And who will shout in our ears *Carpe Diem,* seize the day?

I've seen this done in cancer, lupus, and MS support groups, but never healthy women support groups. I think most people fear being alone more than being in pain.

Honey, I guess there's no use crying because the dear family doctor won't hitch up his buggy and drive over in the dead of night. Medicine is changing. We simply must learn how to get what we need. After that meeting, I was reminded there's power in a group. With all of us together, I feel the wind at my back

Thanks for letting me rattle on. Being able to write my heart out to you all these years has given me more support than you could ever dream!

Write soon.

Love ya,
Barbra Kay

P.S. What is your system for keeping track of medical insurance? The paper work drives me crazy.

TALK TALK TALK

Journal
October 20, 1993

Katherine and her boyfriend Rich drove down from Sacramento in the pouring rain Friday night. After Rich went to sleep in the guest room, Katherine and I flopped across her bed for girl talk. This was the weekend, she told me. Old fashioned and romantic. Rich was going to ask us for her hand in marriage. Katherine planned to visit friends, go shopping, take walks, do anything to give Rich time alone with us.

The next morning I clued Gary in. He stopped his weekend chores and we sat with Rich around the breakfast table talk, talk, talking all Saturday. After prolonged shopping, Katherine grabbed me in the hall. "Did he ask?" I shook my head. She stomped her foot. I whispered that he was nervous, talking a blue streak about everything. I looked into her tearful eyes and squeezed her hand saying,

"Lovey, don't worry. He'll get to it. That guy's in love!"

Well, Saturday night he tried again, and then Sunday at breakfast, then during lunch. "He's going to, Mom. He promised," said Katherine. So Sunday afternoon Katherine went for a long walk, and Gary and I sat in the den listening to Rich talk. After about forty-five minutes I said, "George Richard, do you want to ask us something concerning our daughter?" Like a spring under pressure he gushed out, "Yes! I want to ask for her hand in marriage." Gary's eyes teared up and we both hugged Rich. When Katherine peeked into the den, we shouted congratulations! She had the face of a lily in the sun.

An April wedding! I'm thrilled. For years I'd prayed I'd live long enough to see Katherine married. Now the gift is here! God, help me be well enough to celebrate my daughter and her beloved.

Barbra Goodyear Minar

ODE TO THE PHONE

Journal
January 9, 1994

Oh, phone. How I've hated you this month in bed when you interrupt my needed sleep. When you called me from the shower. When you let some unknown man calling from New York into my bedroom to ask if I wanted to make an investment. But phone, how I love you connecting me with your magic through the skylines to friends. Friends who hear the tears in my voice because I'm sick. Friends who make me laugh. Friends who send courage and prayers through the lines into my ear. Into my soul.

Oh, phone, how I love you saving me steps across town to doctors and pharmacies, auto shops and florists. How I love you letting me hear the voice of my father in Mississippi, telling me he and Hazel are coming to the wedding in spite of his back pain. How I love you for linking me with Katherine so we can talk about white roses and reception music and bridesmaids gifts and satin slippers and the honeymoon food basket and lacy garters and unity candles and the fears of being married forever. Oh, phone, my helper and lifesaver, tonight I put you in your cradle with honor.

WEDDING RIBBONS

March 9, 1994

Dear Katherine Bridelet,
What a whirlwind time. A month from today is your wedding. A month! The little details seem like long colored ribbons blowing in the wind. I run after one and another floats away. Soon they will all be attached to the wedding pole, and the beautiful dance will begin.

This morning as I tied your shower gifts with pink satin, I thought of how many gifts I've wrapped for you. Even as a baby you clapped your pudgy hands and ripped into your packages, tossing the paper over your head. Throughout the years of birthday, Christmas and Valentine's Day surprises, you rewarded me with a smile as big as a quarter moon.

And what a lavish giver you are! You never missed a chance to give gifts you've made or bought. Sweet bride, this time the whole party is for you—all the attention. All the gifts, all the blessings.

My daughter, you are my unexpected treasure. My gift. While we tie down the last of the wedding ribbons, I pray we share the last of your single days with laughter and tenderness. And as we grow as women, may we keep unwrapping the gift of each other.

Mom

JOY

Journal
April 11, 1994

Miracle! I planned. I rested. I asked for help. I planned. I rested. And the wedding, encircled by friends and family, happened.

Jeff walked me to my seat and kissed my cheek. Then Jeff and Steve rolled out the white aisle runner for their sister. The minister waited with the groom and his black tuxedoed groomsmen. The bridesmaids, smiling and pink cheeked, walked down and waited. Music lifted and everyone turned. At the back doors of the church, holding onto Gary, Katherine stood. The daughter from my womb. She stood with two-o'clock sun flooding through her veil, lighting her face, spilling down the satin, lace, and pearls. She stood, and the guests gasped. Suddenly her eyes turned to blue lakes. And as she walked down the aisle, her tears spilled like a shower of stars.

Life, you hold suffering. Suffering presses against me sometimes like smothering smoke, forcing my soul to find meaning or die. I wrestle with the dark enemy, asking God questions. Asking myself questions. On the other side of the fight are the prizes—acceptance and change, wisdom and depth. But, Life, you also hold joy. Joy with her surprising sweetness. Joy's rush fills me until I rock with the pleasure. Until I laugh and cry with the pleasure. The taste of honey intensifies because I've swallowed vinegar. God, You have Your mysterious ways of making us truly human. Living fully means I have to accept the conditions of life. And, today I thank You for the fullness of joy!

WRESTLING DOWN THE BEAR

July 15, 1994

Dearest Jenny,

When you called yesterday, I could hear the tears in your voice. Living with pain is hard enough when you have only yourself to think of, but when you're a wife and mother and you feel all your energy drained away, I know sometimes you feel hopeless. Your doctor saying he didn't think your joint pain was too bad was not helpful. My friend Carolyn was right when she said, "Pain is what the patient says it is!"

Be encouraged, dear heart. I've learned that the challenge of chronic pain is like wrestling down a bear and holding him for the count. You may need a good "wrestling" coach to teach you the techniques for the best control.

I found that learning about pain makes it less scary. Being in pain is both sensory and emotional, so we have to think about both parts. Acute pain is a helpful signal that the body's being damaged. But chronic pain is pain that continues even though there may be little damage done to the body. It can lead to a pain cycle that hurts our well-being. Hurting for days or months on end, we reduce our activities so our muscles weaken. Then we get tired more easily, so we do even less. I think because we can do so little we grow depressed, and when we're depressed we grow more tense and concentrate on the pain. That's when the bear has dragged us into his cave. So we need ways to break out!

Well, here is a list of things I know about and some I've used.

- Exercise
- rest
- acupuncture
- TENS units
- surgery
- hot showers or water therapy
- massage

- ultrasound
- cortisone injections
- visualization
- physical therapy
- imagery
- trigger point
- distraction blocks
- biofeedback
- chiropractors
- medication
- prayer and meditation.

You know Donna Lewis? Well, she went to a pain clinic to find out what's best for her. I'm sure she'll share her experience. Maybe you could consider going, too.

Different things work for me for different pain problems. I know there's a strong psychological part to this. The more afraid I get, the worse the pain gets. I took some relaxation sessions learning how to breathe and relax all the major muscles. Also, I found out that distraction helps me. When my attention is focused on the pain, it's worse. I try to distract myself by visiting with someone, seeing a good movie (funny is best), reading or writing. I've used imagery (learned this in the dentist chair). In my imagination I see myself walking with my dog under the arch of elm trees along the road in Briarwood Ranch. Or sometimes I will try to solve a problem or make up a fantasy about going to an enchanted island. Sometimes I need medication.

It seems funny, but I've found what I say to myself about the pain makes a difference. Exaggerating the pain or saying "I can't stand this," "This is the worse pain I've ever had," "I can never do anything fun again," all makes me more depressed and unable to cope.

I try (and sometimes it's a tremendous effort) to tell myself:
- Barbra, the pain *will* end. You can make it.
- *Stop* thinking negatively.
- Breathe deeply. Relax

Walking Into The Wind   185

- Barbra, distract yourself. Do something.

Jenny, love, I'm so sad you have to deal with this constant pain. But there is hope! It may be the toughest challenge you ever face. But the pain is treatable! Learn some techniques to wrestle that bear, and you'll be more in charge and feel more positive. What a warrior you are! It's a sign you are really healthy even in the battle!

Blessings,
Barbra

P.S. Keep calling! Reaching out is *extremely* important. And share the things you discover with *me*. This old dog can always learn a few new tricks. Kiss Mark and beautiful Sarah for me!

Barbra Goodyear Minar

RUNNING AWAY

December 12, 1994

Dear Frances,

Oh, honey, was I glad to hear your Thanksgiving went so well because you asked your family to share the load. Now here we are launching into Christmas. And (you'll love this) I had planned to send my packages out last Tuesday to beat the pressure and crowds. I was in a hurry. You know the trap. To accomplish a lot, better move faster, because you're already tired.

Well, I planned to let my dog ride to the post office, but when I let Happy outside, instead of jumping in the car, she trotted into the front yard, across the drive into our neighbor's lawn whipping her tail in the wind. Yelling in my loudest fishwife voice, I hurried next door, but she broke into a run and vanished into the brush-covered creek. That lab! Since she was a pup she'd only be confined so long. Then pouf—she was off on an adventure alone. She hides herself in shrubs, under porches, behind trees—anywhere to remain free. Now after eleven years of hunting her down without success, I've learned to let her go. Eventually the old girl always comes back, muddy and smelly, blinking her brown eyes and nosing me with her silver muzzle.

Standing there, swinging the car keys and growling under my breath, I stared after her with a longing in my chest. And Frances, I realized *I* needed to run away and maybe even come back a little muddy. But there was so much to be done. Never mind, I told myself. Learn from your dog!

So, I drove to the beach overcast and chilly. Wrapped in a blanket I sat on the beach losing myself in the sea life. Sitting on a rock, my bare feet buried in the wet sand, I let ocean music sing to my soul. Christmas. Christmas. It would be what it would be. The most important thing for me was to be present with my people. My family. My friends. My God. I watched gray gulls sky floating on the wind currents. And I felt the holiday details lift off my shoulders like sea birds.

When I got home all sandy and tired, there was that muddy, scoundrel dog sleeping on her back in the sun, all four feet in the air, as happy as I was.

Merry Christmas, my dear friend. May your New Year be filled with a little sky floating and private moments of wonder.

Love,
Barbra Kay

WISDOM OF THE NINETIES

Journal
January 13, 1995

Yesterday Ruth had a birthday. She was ninety. I wanted to go over, but I didn't have much energy after paying the bills, trying to get a manuscript ready to mail, doing a load of wash. No matter how I push I'm always behind.

After a short nap, I pulled myself together and hurried to her apartment. I knocked on her door, holding three pink balloons. She opened it wide, as if she'd been standing there waiting. "I don't want those," she barked from her walker. "Give them to some kid." I laughed and told Ruth we were all kids at heart. "No," she said. "I'm no kid. I'm older than dirt. Come on." She scooted ahead of me, pushing her walker with its bright yellow tennis balls on the front legs, letting me follow with the balloons. I told her she looked spiffy in her red jacket. "I get it out every birthday. If I forget next year, you'll know I've lost my mind for sure. Promise to shoot me." I laughed. Ruth's a rascal.

It took us a long time to make the walk to the cheerful dining room of the Solvang Lutheran Home. Once a month the birthdays are celebrated with a special afternoon party—cake, ice cream, the works. All the residents come and are served by volunteers. And a wonderful young woman, Suzanne, plays the piano and sings. Suzanne smiled like sunshine. "Ruth, how lucky can you be! The party falls right on your birthday." Grumbling, Ruth just kept pushing her walker until she found her table and sat down. "What you gonna do with those fool balloons," she looked at me and adjusted her glasses. "You might as well tie them on my chair." "Might as well," I said. It was hard to keep a straight face.

Soon Emma and Millie hung their canes on the chair backs and joined our table. I asked Ruth about the first birthday she could remember. She told about her tenth birthday when her daddy borrowed a big roan horse for her to ride the whole day. She told about the picnic with her folks down by the creek and taking that horse through the cold stream while her daddy stood on the bank and shouted directions. "He was scared, I think. But he let me go. I was in such a hurry to grow big and have my own horse. Don't know what the hurry was all about."

While we ate more cake and sipped more coffee, Millie and Emma, also in their nineties, exchanged memories with Ruth. I heard wisdom—how these women accepted both shining days and howling storms. They've learned to wait until the wind dies down. They've learned how to go on. Before I knew it, the afternoon slipped away. As I walked to my car, I felt relaxed, like I'd been on a mini-vacation. No one cared if I got everything done, no one cared if I forgot things, no one cared if I dawdled. Their world had slowed down, and it is exactly the right speed for me. Yeah! What's the hurry.

Barbra Goodyear Minar

THE GIFT OF THE MARK

Journal
April 12, 1995

I've been thinking about these lesions on my left cheek. For years I've searched the drug store shelves for something to cover the marks—bottles and jars of lotions and potions and brown, green, and pink makeup. Saleswomen leaning across glass counters patting me with various shades of cover up and powders. The effect looked artificial, but without makeup the three red circles are always visible. Well, that's not entirely true. Sometimes they fade into white rings until the sun, a fever, or a lupus flare wakes them. Then they boil up hot and red like burns from a dashboard cigarette lighter. When I feel the burning, my hand flies to my cheek like an involuntary sigh to hide the marks.

Last month I went to lunch at Side's Street Cafe with a few women. We were laughing and talking over our Chinese chicken salads when Donna and Elaine's breezy conversation turned into a stormy disagreement. Their eyes narrowed and snapped as the argument escalated. Truth, standing tall in his high topped hat, was poked and bent into a pretzel man. My cheek began to burn.

The two women moved apart as their icy words clinked around the table. "So, Barbra," Elaine turned to me. "Don't you think Donna's off track?" They were both off track, and I wanted to make tracks and get out of there. But mumbling a few words, I tried to play peacemaker. My cheek felt like it was on fire. Pushing back my chair, I headed for the bathroom to splash cold water on my face. Sure enough. Staring back at me from the mirror were three bright red welts. Embarrassed, I dabbed my cheek with powder. The quarrel was stressful enough. Why did I have to deal with this?

It took a few days, but the lesions cooled off until two weeks ago when I met Paul and Donald at the Coffee Bean. I knew Paul liked to joke around, but when he and Donald started telling radical political jokes, I felt uncomfortable. I interrupted their guffaws, asking for ideas about helping a mutual friend. Back to the jokes. Now they were even worse! My face heated up. I felt the lesions puffing out. I held my ice tea glass against my blistering cheek. For the next twenty minutes I listened to a monster merry-go-round of words.

Now, I've noticed that if Gary and I have a disagreement, the marks don't get red. If I'm working something out with a friend, they don't get red. They appear when I feel caught, a cat cornered by a barking dog. Health is listening to my body—so maybe the marks I've hated are a signal. A gift. They're announcing in their hot fierce way I need to protect myself. The next time the lesions talk to me I'm going to honor their voice. "Oh, so sorry," I'll say. "I have to be going. My cheek's on fire."

I'M FEELIN' FINE AND OTHER LITTLE LIES

July 1995

Dear Jenny,

You asked me yesterday me if I got irritated when every person I meet asks, "How are you feeling?" I gave you a quick "no," but in thinking about it I see that's not true.

"How are you feeling?" It came to me from Mollie and Joe at the church Sunday morning, Janie Tillman at the bank on Monday, Jerry Ross at Nielsen's Market on Tuesday—"How are you feeling? How are you feeling?"

I'm sure people are trying to connect, to care, but it stops deeper communication. I get sick of talking about my illness—about me. Probably everyone else is sick of it, too, especially Gary who hears my response over and over. "Fine. I'm fine." Now that's pretty silly if I have swollen eyes and I'm clutching the grocery cart to stand up. "How are you feeling?" Sometimes I *want* to shout, "AWFUL AND I DON'T WANT TO TALK ABOUT IT!" What a dilemma. Why am I confused about this? It's because I want to have natural connection and real conversation. "How do you feel?" Well, now that you've asked, I feel like fly fishing in Colorado, I feel like traveling to London to see Cats, I feel like going swimming in the nude, I feel like singing La Boheme . . . la la la LAAAA."

All kidding aside, I try to remember people are reaching out, but I am resisting being identified as "the poor sick girl." I am more than my body. I am *me* with a million other things going on in my soul worth talking about. So when Mollie and Joe ask "How are you feeling?" I've learned to smile and say "How are *you?*" And, dear heart, their stories tumble out. It works every time.

Blessings,
Barbra

HEADSTRONG

Journal
December 29, 1995

This morning I glanced through the Sunday <u>Santa Barbara News-Press</u> and a picture on page three stalled my mind. I clipped out the article and put it on my desk. Among a circle of bald heads crowded together in a huddle, two shining faces smile up at the camera. The caption read:

"Basketball squad of sixth-graders from Cambridge, Minnesota, after they shaved their heads to show support for their friend and teammate, Kane Nelson. Kane was undergoing chemotherapy treatment for leukemia in a Minneapolis hospital."

Staring at the eleven bald boys, I could hear the kids asking, "Wasn't Kane playing with us just two weeks ago? And later didn't he go with us to the movies? Did you guys know he was that sick? Did you know he's taking chemotherapy and losing all his hair. Gosh! Do you think he might even—die?"

I wonder which boy said, "Hey, what if we shaved our heads? You know, the whole team. We'll be like Kane." I wish I could have been there when the hearts of the youngsters caught fire with the idea. I can imagine the boys saying, "Hey, coach, we wanna shave our heads for Kane." Each one had to face his parents. "Hey, Mom, I wanna shave my head for Kane." Each one stood in front of a mirror. "Hey, I'm not sure I wanna do this. I'm gonna look like a geek."

Together they probably went to the local barber shop where the barbers donated the shaves, and eleven young lions watched each other lose their manes. That night some of them probably took a ribbing from their sisters and went to bed with stocking caps on their nude heads to keep from freezing. But I know each one felt proud. And now as they shoot together on the court, they can look at each other and know they connected with their friend. After the shave these boys will be different.

Barbra Goodyear Minar

The're all richer, more sensitive young men who understand the power of caring and the power of community. These will be the men of our future. Men who can stand in a storm. Surely I'm richer, too, because they shaved their heads.

JUDY'S SOUP

Journal
January 8, 1996

I'm alone. Lying in bed like a sack of potatoes. My body's quiet. But my mind's like an egg beater whipping together writing paper, orange juice, cleaning rags, left-over mashed potatoes, paper clips, thank-you notes and bills. My to-do-first-of-the-year list is as long as some books I've read. But I'm too weak to even brush my teeth.

Judy phoned. "I'm coming with dinner," she said firmly and drove her blue van into my driveway exactly at 5:30 p.m. I heard her dry cough as she got out of her car. I opened the back door. Gripping her arm crutches, her disability vanished as she moved her delicate body to the back porch while magically manipulating a container steaming with chicken and dumplings. "You should be in bed." Her voice was like a scolding wind. Studying me with squinting blue eyes through a white fringe of bangs, her forehead pleated. She frowned. I liked it. Her mothering. Her loving sternness. "The dumpling are still cooking from the heat," she said. "My mother's recipe." I backed away from her thin frame with a warning not to catch my flu.

"No, no, don't worry about me." She shook her head and gave an impish smile. "I know what you need! This is better for you than chicken soup. Real healing ingredients. Now get into bed!"

Judy's angel face is imprinted on my mind as I spoon her chicken dumplings and bravery into my mouth. Ah, heavenly custard.

Barbra Goodyear Minar

LIGHT EXPLOSION

Journal
February 10, 1996

About seven this morning I was sipping apple spice tea and watching a fight at the bird feeder when the phone rang. "Mom?" After three months of silence, it was Jeff. "Mom, are you sitting down?" My tea turned bitter. My stomach cramped. Like electricity running down a line, thoughts of Jeff's emergency history blitzed through me, and my cheek blistered up. "After all your prayers, Mom, I wanted to tell you first."

I held on to the edge of the kitchen table as he told a story of being alone in a cheap hotel room after over-dosing from drugs and alcohol. No money, no friends, he lay in the dark across a filthy bed. No hope. He waited for death.

"A light," he said, "an intense light came through the ceiling and all around me." Here, into this hell came God. God loved him. Jeff's words were flowing over me like a warm wind scented with lavender. Loved him. The words flowed into me like a transfusion.

Jeff took a deep breath, and with boy-like energy, his words tumbled out. "I felt this Presence. This Power. And I knew with God I can do anything. Mom, I gave God control of my life."

I was crying by then. An eternal waterfall stored in my underground river found its way out and over the cliff. The water I stored when I saw some woman's healthy son working hard stocking shelves at Roeser's Pharmacy, a strong boy riding a mountain bike with friends up Figueroa Mountain Road or going to the Saturday night movies with his special girl. The water I stored when I read about a young man Jeff's age graduating from college or getting married. I stored all the tears in my river. Now I cried. For the answer to my groaning beyond words, for the answer to prayers that had stayed fastened to my tongue for nineteen years. For the prayers of Jeff's father, grandmother, and grandfather. For the prayers of his sister and brother. For the prayers of countless friends and prayer circles. For the prayers of recovering drug

MINA

users and strangers who heard my plea and carried him into the spiritual realm for holy help. I cried from joy bursting my frame.

How often I'd wondered if I would ever know my son. Really know him as a man. Sane and in his right mind. What happened to the chubby baby who pushed away from my breast to pat my cheek and coo? The toddler who talked a blue streak and wore his cowboy hat in the bathtub? The young boy who bloodied Jimmy Ladner's nose to protect his little sister? Drugs stole him away. Stole him from his trumpet and drums. Stole him from algebra and history. Stole him from tennis and wrestling. Stole him from Boy Scouts and 4-H. Stole him from his father. His brother and sister. From me. And worst of all, stole him from himself. He was stolen from life; he was kidnapped by a demon.

The demon imprisoned him in a labyrinth of the Dark. And Jeff couldn't read the map of escape. He was blind. No matter how many candles anyone lit for him, he couldn't see the way out. His rescue required a miracle. A Light explosion.

Oh, God! Thank you for your mercy. I am singing. I am dancing. I am shouting for joy. My son was lost, and now he is found. And I am alive to see this day. I will get to know the man you made.

Barbra Goodyear Minar

A TENT TO REST IN

Journal
July 21, 1996

I wasn't strong enough to make the trip to Portland alone. When I asked Steve for help, he said he'd love to go see Jeff with me. Love to. And so I began the resting. The resting. The resting. And packing. All the medications and vitamins I might possibly need. So often our family had waded into darkness when we visited Jeff. This time we had our eyes full of light and hope.

There was a baking wind at 105 degrees when we arrived. Heat smothered my body, and I was drained. I so wanted to be well for these few days. Arriving at the motel Jeff had arranged, I flopped on my bed while Steven called his brother. In five minutes he knocked on our door. "Hi Mom!" Tall. He stood straight and tall. Dark curly hair and mustache trimmed short. Calm hazel eyes looked into my center, washing me with wonder. Jeff hugged me, gathering me into the mix of his clean smelling hair and Old Spice, and I let my wet face rest against him. My deep fatigue drained away.

Steve slapped him on the back. "Looking good, bro!" Then he threw his arms around us making a tent. A tent of bodies and blood and hearts and history. A tent to start out from again.

We met Jeff's love. His Barbara. And for the next few days we explored the area together, driving first to the Pacific. As Jeff walked barefoot along flat wide beach at Seaside, I watched him lift his face and arms to the sun and then stoop to write huge love messages to Barbara in the sand. The next day, driving inland along the Columbia River to the Cascade Locks, Jeff pointed out a fish hatchery. I watched the brothers splash each other like young boys as they fed and petted the huge breeding salmon.

The last morning exploring Portland, we went to see the Imperial Tombs of China at the Portland Art Museum. Like a man whose blindfold had been just ripped away, Jeff studied the ancient terra-cotta warriors and walked around the case holding the Ming dragon and phoe-

MINA

nix gold, dazzling with jewels and blue kingfisher bird feathers. In the middle of the exhibit Jeff grabbed my hand. "Mom, I'm so thankful—to be alive!"

The four days were filled with talking and hugging and laughing and comfortable silences. The silence that comes with love speaking without words. Speaking from skin to skin. I came daring to hope the cyclone was over. I found blessed peace. I came daring to hope improvement was evident. I came and found a miracle!

THE SINGER

November 17, 1996

Dear Jenny,

When you told me about little Sarah's eye problem last week, I wanted to comfort you; say something helpful, but my mouth seemed full of feathers. How I wished I could give you magic words that would heal this heartache. And I know you're asking, isn't my lupus enough? Why this? Why now? Why my daughter? Oh, Jenny, there isn't an answer to these questions. Life seems to surprise us with both gifts and losses. Many people have the illusion that if we follow the right map and stay on the road, we can keep all windstorms from our life. We can stay in control, receive the gifts and avoid the pain. But that's not the way of the journey.

In the ache of our losses, sometimes there are gifts. When our road's been washed out and our map's obsolete—when we stand still in the dark calling for direction, God comes close to us. He gifts us with Himself. Pain brings us into the present moment and we learn that's where life is. We stop rushing and look in the eyes of our children. We let the kitten sleep on our chest. We laugh when our friend tells a funny story. We touch the soft cheek of the grandmother. We stop and drink in life. I pray you and Mark will look for gifts as you help walk Sarah through the frustrations. God won't disappoint you.

Last May, when I felt very undone by my fatigue, I wrote this little story in my journal.

Once there was a crippled girl who sat by the gate of her village. Every day she sat and sang about her gifts. Gifts of a red bird swooping overhead, gifts of the scent from the locust tree, gifts of thunder speaking from the windy sky. People walked by and listened to her songs. People walked by and left a potato or onion or sometimes a bit of meat in her bowl. And every night the girl lifted her voice, thanking God for her soup. The next morning she would sing once more about the gift of rain washing her face, the gift of the baby sleeping in his mother's arms, the gift of pinks and orange from the setting sun. Through the years the people walked by and listened and smiled and sometimes cried. The people walked by and left a potato or onion or sometimes a bit of meat in her bowl. Time passed, and one morning a village boy found a gray haired woman slumped by the gate. "The old cripple's dead!" he shouted. "No, no," whispered the people, touching her bowl. "The singer. The singer."

Cry, my dear heart, but learn to sing in the midst of rain and the sun, and you will help Sarah become a singer.

I love you all,
Barbra

THE GIFT IN THE SHADOW

Journal
January 6, 1997

I'm growing old. I passed by the light-struck mirror in the hall and saw a silver haired girl with the face of a grandmother. I stood transfixed, feeling ageless under the etched lines on my cheeks and chin. I stood there surprised! I have lived long enough to grow old.

I thank God for the models in my life. People like Melva Wickman who at eighty-six years puts in her contact lens, delicately makes up her beautiful face and goes to a concert or play. "Have you read this book?" she'll say. "Sorry you couldn't get me. I was just counseling some girls from Westmont College. When can we go out to lunch?" Melva continued giving Christian retreats around the country until two years ago. People flock to her for wisdom and truth because she's as transparent and reflective as a piece of crystal. I would sit at her feet, but she insists we sit elbow to elbow like good friends.

And Laura Wilkening at eighty-five wearing purple leotards and a purple coat she wove. Her white hair like a crown, she walks full of grace through her lush garden, showing me new rose bushes and complaining she can't work on her knees as long as she used to. She kisses and hugs her friends with great abandon and her encouraging words land on us like butterflies. When I told her I wanted to write poetry, Laura's smile lifted her blushing cheeks and she clapped her hands saying, "Good for you. Good for you." Still learning and traveling and weaving and collecting art, she is completely herself. She encourages my becoming.

These women work around their ailing bodies. When they must, they see the doctor, go to bed and take their herbs and pills. And they live with pain. And they live with gratefulness.

I am old. The wind has blown me over many times and yet I find I'm still here. I am learning how to walk into the wind. My older friends now live in the shadow of death. It's the edge of the shadow that intensifies life. Perhaps this shadow that came at twenty has offered a great gift to me all these years. The gift of claiming my days with awe. With wonder. And stretching towards the mysterious God who has tomorrow waiting in another kingdom.

EVERYTHING I NEED IS HERE

Journal
November 26, 1997

Tomorrow is Thanksgiving, and so today I mended the hole in Gram Dupuy's old lace tablecloth. I pulled the silver chest from under the couch and made black marks on the gray cloth as I polished the spoons. I chopped the onions and apples on the scarred wooden board for the dressing. I floured the counter and kneaded the bread. I let it rise. I punched it down. I let it rise. I baked the bread. I baked the bread.

More than once I grieved for my dreams of greatness. If only I had been brilliant, I could have been a pediatrician or botany professor. If only I had more courage and more strength, I could have climbed Kilimanjaro or sailed to the Greek Islands. If only I hadn't married so young, I could have worked for the Peace Corps. If only I hadn't been sick, I could have done something more meaningful with my life. I could have left my imprint. Made the world a better place. But as I watch the bread rise on my counter, I know that all I need is here. Here I have great things to do. I have gifts to give away.

What life! Life and health in the apples and the onions. Life and health in mending holes and shining silver. Life and health in the bread that feeds my family. The love that waters my family and makes story.

I belong in this simple holy place.
Concealed in the simple
is greatness.

Barbra Goodyear Minar

EPILOGUE

STRIPPING OFF SKINS

As Gary and I drove along the ocean toward Pismo Beach, the gray February afternoon reminded me that God wraps our future in a fog. Much to my surprise I will be sixty next summer. Our three children are married to their best friends. Three grandsons bring us joy; a granddaughter will grace us this spring. In June, Gary and I will celebrate our fortieth anniversary. All this occurred as I stumbled and walked through each day. Crying days and laughing days mixed with the rough and the smooth. Along the way I unwrapped living-gifts.

When Gary pulled into the parking lot of the Monarch Butterfly Refuge, I saw few visitors. We walked the short distance through rain sprinkles to the thick leaf carpet of the sanctuary. Breathing the unmistakable pungent fragrance, I squinted up into the tall eucalyptus trees. Fluttering under the tree limbs were several brilliant orange and black patterned butterflies, but not in the abundance I expected. These fragile creatures had traveled over the Sierras and west of the Rockies from as far away as Canada to winter here from October through February. Maybe only a few survived this year. The rain came down harder, breaking through the tree-shelter. Disappointed, I snapped open my umbrella and decided to leave. A sudden gust of wind gave the tree branches a toss.

"There they are," said a young man, handing me his binoculars. "Aren't they incredible!" I focused though the lens. Concealed in the trees were huge clusters of butterflies. With their delicate wings closed, the butterflies hid their colors, blending into the eucalyptus leaves. Protected from the wind and rain, they rested,

MINA

perfectly camouflaged, overlapping each other like tiny shingles. As my eyes adjusted to their presence, I walked the path discovering thousands and thousands of Monarchs in the grove. Sitting on a wooden bench, I gazed at the hidden magic.

A woman pointed at a monarch near our feet and told me they'd fly north to lay their eggs. "But before a caterpillar is in its chrysalis and changes into a butterfly, it sheds its skin four times. They're amazing!"

I have heard the story of the chrysalis and the miraculous emergence of the butterfly many times. But never the loss of four skins in the process. Standing in the midst of these exquisite creatures, I wondered about our human growth from birth to death. Perhaps during our journeys pain strips off our old skins because we are still becoming. Becoming aware. Becoming simpler. Becoming thankful. One day there will be no more tears. As the mystery unfolds, we will emerge into the free eternal beings God intends. The fog will lift. We will fly with the wind.

Barbra Goodyear Minar

NOTES

1. Isaiah 57:10, *Revised Standard Version of the Bible.*
2. Tournier, Paul, *The Meaning of Persons* (San Francisco: Harper & Row, 1957), p. 83.
3. Psalm 30:11-12, *Revised Standard Version of the Bible.*
4. Tim Hansel, *You Gotta Keep Dancin',* (Elgin, Il: David C. Cook Publishing Company, 1985), p.37.
5. Psalm 31:24, *Revised Standard Version of the Bible.*
6. Scott Peck, *The Road Less Traveled,* (New York: Simon & Schuster, 1978), p. 15.
7. Ted B.Engstrom, *The Pursuit of Excellence,* (Grand Rapids, Michigan: Zondervan, 1982), p. 88-89.
8. Madeline L'Engle, *Walking on Water,* (Wheaton, Il:Harold Shaw Publisher,1980), p.72.
9. Einstein, "What I Believe," *Forum,* October 1930.
10. Guilbert, Charles Mortimer, *The Book of Common Prayer,* (The Church Hymnal Corporation and Seabury Press, 1977), p.461.

MINA